Royal Society of Medicine Services Limited

International Congress and Symposium Series

Editor-in-Chief: H. J. C. L'Etang

Number 97

Recent advances in the treatment of urinary tract infections

Proceedings of a Symposium sponsored by Norwich Eaton Pharmaceuticals, Inc., and held at the Academic Medical Centre, Amsterdam, on 18 September 1985

Royal Society of Medicine Services Limited

International Congress and Symposium Series

Number 97

Recent advances in the treatment of urinary tract infections

Edited by

F. H. SCHRÖDER

1985

Published by

ROYAL SOCIETY OF MEDICINE SERVICES LIMITED
1 Wimpole Street, London W1M 8AE

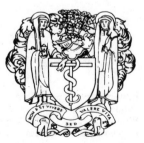

ROYAL SOCIETY OF MEDICINE SERVICES LIMITED
1 Wimpole Street, London W1M 8AE

Distributed by

OXFORD UNIVERSITY PRESS
Walton Street, Oxford OX2 6DP

London   New York   Toronto
Delhi   Bombay   Calcutta   Madras   Karachi
Kuala Lumpur   Singapore   Hong Kong   Tokyo
Nairobi   Dar es Salaam   Cape Town
Melbourne   Auckland

and associated companies in
Beirut   Berlin   Ibadan   Mexico City   Nicosia

Oxford is a trade mark of Oxford University Press
Copyright © 1985 by

ROYAL SOCIETY OF MEDICINE SERVICES LIMITED

These proceedings are published by Royal Society of Medicine Services Ltd with financial support from the sponsor. The contributors are responsible for the scientific content and for the views expressed, which are not necessarily those of the sponsor, of the editor of the series or of the volume, of the Royal Society of Medicine or of Royal Society of Medicine Services Ltd. Distribution has been in accordance with the wishes of the sponsor but a copy is available to any Fellow of the Society at a privileged price.

British Library Cataloguing in Publication Data
Recent advances in the treatment of urinary
    tract infections. — (International congress
    and symposium series; no. 97)
    1. Urinary organs — Disease — Chemotherapy
    I. Schröder, F. H.   II. Series
    615'.761   RC901.7.C4

ISBN 0-905958-24-1

Editorial assistance: S. A. L. Filcek, Professional Postgraduate Services Ltd, Sunderland House, Sunderland Street, Macclesfield, Cheshire SK11 6JF
Phototypeset by Dobbie Typesetting Service, Plymouth, Devon
Printed in Great Britain at the University Press, Oxford

Contributors

Editor

Professor F. H. Schröder
> Department of Urology, Faculty of Medicine, Erasmus University, Dr Molewaterplein 50, 3015 GE Rotterdam, The Netherlands

Dr I. Bollgren
> Assistant Professor of Paediatrics, Karolinska Institute, Sachsska Children's Hospital, Sachsska Barnsjukhuset, Sachsgaten 1, 10064 Stockholm, Sweden

Professor W. Brumfitt
> Professor and Head of Department of Medical Microbiology and Consultant in Charge of Urinary Infection Clinic, The Royal Free Hospital, Pond Street, Hampstead, London NW3 2QG, UK

Professor J. N. Corriere Jr
> Professor and Director, Division of Urology, University of Texas Health Science Centre, 6431 Fannin, Suite 6018, Texas Medical Center, Houston, Texas 77030, USA

Professor P. F. D'Arcy
> Head of Department and Dean, Faculty of Science, Department of Pharmacy, Medical Biology Centre, The Queen's University of Belfast, 97 Lisburn Road, Belfast, Northern Ireland, UK

Dr J. M. T. Hamilton-Miller
> Urinary Infection Clinic, The Royal Free Hospital, Pond Street, Hampstead, London NW3 2QG, UK

Professor P. J. Whalley
> Department of Obstetrics and Gynecology, Texas Health Science Center, 5323 Harry Hines Boulevard, Dallas, Texas 75235, USA

Contents

Foreword

This volume presents the proceedings of a symposium on recent advances in the treatment of urinary tract infections (UTIs). The symposium took place in Amsterdam in September 1985 and was held as a satellite meeting to the Second European Meeting on Urological Endoscopy, organized under the auspices of the Departments of Urology at the Universities of Amsterdam, Leiden and Nijmegen, the Netherlands, in association with The Institute of Urology, London, UK.

The symposium was convened in order to assess the parameters against which a drug therapy for UTIs should be measured, with special reference to nitrofurantoin. The meeting has been structured to deal in turn with each of these points and to assess the profile of nitrofurantoin with reference to the features of the 'ideal' drug for the treatment of UTI:

Urinary tract specificity;

Lack of development of resistance to therapy;

Effectiveness in a wide range of patients;

Safety of use during pregnancy;

Minimum of adverse effects, reactions and interactions with other therapies.

A further point to note is that urinary tract infection should not be regarded as a single disease entity: it is a spectrum of diseases and, as such, some antibacterial agents may be more suitable than others in the treatment of various types of infection.

Many different classes of drugs—sulphonamides, penicillins, nitrofurantoin, cephalosporins, quinolones etc—have been introduced in the past 50 or so years that make up the 'antibiotic era'. Some have fallen into disfavour and disuse owing to the emergence of resistance and adverse safety profiles. Nitrofurantoin, introduced 30 years ago, has, however, maintained a good profile against the parameters outlined above, as will be seen in the following chapters, and thus remains one of the most widely used therapies for the treatment of UTI.

Fritz H. Schröder
Rotterdam
September 1985

Introduction:
Comments on urinary tract infections

F. H. SCHRÖDER

*Department of Urology, Erasmus University,
Rotterdam, The Netherlands*

Urinary tract infection (UTI) is one of the most common disease entities dealt with by urologists, general practitioners and all other members of the medical profession. The urologist more frequently than others is confronted with UTI, because it is his task to deal with many of the conditions that are known to promote UTIs. Also, the urological diagnostic work-up and urological management of disease frequently necessitate the invasion of the urinary tract, which may be complicated by the introduction of bacteria. Furthermore, it is the role of the urologist to diagnose and deal with UTIs which are complicated by promoting factors. For these obvious reasons, the urologist must be equipped with detailed knowledge about all aspects of UTIs.

The field of UTIs has been developing very quickly during recent years. It has become possible to detect new host factors, which may explain why some individuals without any urological predisposing factors are susceptible to UTIs, by exploring further the phenomenon of bacterial adherence to epithelial cells of the urinary tract. At the same time, new bacterial factors have been detected which can explain the virulence of some bacterial strains — as opposed to others — in causing UTIs. Such new developments, together with the continuous development of new drugs and new therapeutic principles, give continuous fascination to scientists and clinicians for the field of urology. These developments have also resulted in the necessity of continuous efforts in postgraduate training for those professionals who have to deal with this complex disease entity in their daily practice.

Before reviewing some of the features of UTIs, for a better understanding, it is necessary to introduce some definitions. A simple clinical classification of UTIs is

Table 1

Clinical classification of UTI

Asymptomatic bacteriuria
Uncomplicated, symptomatic UTI
Complicated UTI
 (symptomatic or asymptomatic)

Recent advances in the treatment of urinary tract infections, edited by F. H. Schröder, 1985: Royal Society of Medicine Services International Congress and Symposium Series No. 97, published by Royal Society of Medicine Services Limited.

given in Table 1. Asymptomatic bacteriuria is found on routine bacteriological examination of urine. Bacteriuria is considered significant if more than 100 000 bacteria per cm^3 are found (1). Uncomplicated symptomatic UTIs, usually with symptoms of cystitis, are diagnosed by the presence of a significant symptomatic bacteriuria in the absence of abnormal urological findings. In complicated UTIs, which may be symptomatic or asymptomatic, significant bacteriuria is accompanied by abnormalities of the urinary tract, which are considered to be promoting factors.

Obviously, the goal of treatment of UTIs is the eradication of bacteria and their long-term prevention. In order to judge upon the failure of treatment, it is necessary to classify the different types of recurrences that may be observed. A summary is given in Table 2. *Recurrence* is defined as significant bacteriuria with or without symptoms. *Treatment failure* is commonly defined as persistence of the UTI with the same causative organism. *Relapse* indicates recurrence of UTI with the same organism. The two episodes are separated by an interval during which no significant bacteriuria and no symptoms are found. A *reinfection* is characterized by the occurrence of significant bacteriuria caused by a new organism with or without a disease-free interval.

Table 2

'Recurrence' of UTI: definitions

Treatment failure — persistence of infection with same organism
Relapse — recurrence of UTI with same organism
Reinfection — a new infection with a different organism, with or without disease-free interval

Incidence and natural history of UTIs

The incidence and prevalence of UTIs are known from the studies of open populations which have been published by several authors (2,3).

In the series of studies by Haag and Valkenburg (2,4), an open population of children and adults was screened. In these reports, the prevalence of bacteriuria in females varied between $0 \cdot 5$ and 10%. The higher prevalence was found in older age groups. In males there was an overall prevalence of bacteriuria of 2%. All 200 individuals showing significant bacteriuria were studied urologically. In 40% of these cases, some urological abnormalities of the upper or lower tract were found. Insufficient emptying of the upper or lower tract was identified as a predisposing factor. In the open population, a prevalence of radiological signs of pyelonephritis was found in 14%. In patients who had been previously treated for UTIs the prevalence was 35%. Very few of the detected urological abnormalities required treatment (4).

The annual incidence of cystitis in the population studied by Valkenburg (4) was 1–2%. Over the whole study period, the prevalence of symptoms of cystitis was 10% in children below the age of 10 and 50% in older women. The prevalence of pyelonephritic changes ranged from 2 to 20% in women and from 1 to 4% in men. Loss of renal function was seen in one of 3000 individuals in the open population. It was calculated that mortality of renal disease in The Netherlands amounts to one per 100 000 inhabitants per year (4).

Important information concerning the natural history of untreated bacteriuria was produced by Haag's and Valkenburg's studies (2,4). In slightly more than 40% of patients, bacteria disappeared spontaneously from the urinary tract within 1 year. About 10% developed symptoms, whilst the remaining significant bacteriurias remained asymptomatic. Within 1 year, 40% showed a change of the bacterial flora.

The study also showed a high incidence of urological abnormalities with the presence of asymptomatic bacteriuria. It remains doubtful, however, whether this correlation indicates a positive relation between urological abnormalities and the presence of bacteriuria. Significant bacteriuria is also found in large numbers of individuals, who, on urological examinations, are found not to have anatomical defects. Since UTI is the parameter used for screening, it remains unknown how many urological abnormalities exist without associated UTI. Daily practice shows that this is frequently the case. The question as to whether and which type of urological abnormalities do in fact cause UTI can only be answered by the study of open populations using other screening tests, such as ultrasound studies of the kidney and the bladder or by prospective longitudinal studies in which the effect of surgical treatment is compared with the effect of antibacterial treatment. Until such evidence is produced, our knowledge about the correlation of urological abnormalities with bacteriuria will remain patchy.

The authors conclude from their studies (2,4) that screening for bacteriuria and treatment of asymptomatic bacteriuria are not necessary.

Kunin (3) studied a large population of schoolchildren and identified 156 girls with significant persistent bacteriuria. These children were treated with short antibiotic courses and followed over long periods of time. For the indication of treatment in this series, it did not matter whether bacteriuria was symptomatic or asymptomatic. This study, which covered the time from 1960 through 1962, produced important information on the recurrence of bacteriuria after treatment. Kunin showed that 10 days of treatment with sulphonamide 'cured' 20–25% of asymptomatic or symptomatic bacteriurias. Of the 126 white girls, 50% showed recurrences within 1 year, and 75–80% showed recurrences within 3 years. If the time between recurrences was very short, more frequent recurrences were observed. Treatment of recurrences again led to the 'cure' of similar proportions of patients. This led to the description of a logarithmic decay curve for the incidence of recurrences, which correlated markedly with age. It is interesting to note that, in Kunin's study (3), the presence or absence of reflux did not have any significant impact on recurrence rates. Unfortunately, it is not known whether the logarithmic decrease of the recurrence rate with age would also occur in an untreated population. However, the general decrease of bacteriuria in children with age, also observed by Kunin in children older than 15 years, may suggest this.

Pathogenesis of UTI

In discussing the pathogenesis of UTIs, it is important to consider separately those factors that *per se* lead to bacteriuria and those factors that lead to organ damage by UTI. A number of conditions and risk factors are clearly identifiable by a higher incidence of symptomatic UTIs, which may result in damage of the kidneys or the urinary tract; these are summarized in Table 3. Since it is well established that bacteria found in the urinary tract are identical to those found in the gastrointestinal tract of the same host, risk factors must in some way promote the penetration of such bacteria from the anal area into the urinary tract. The work by Stamey and his group (5), showing colonization by bacterial flora of the area of the external meatus of the urethra in females by bacteria in some individuals and not in others, represents

Table 3

Risk factors in UTI

Childhood
Pregnancy
Urological abnormalities:
    trauma and foreign bodies
Bacterial adherence
    (presence of receptors for P-fimbriae)

Table 4

Model of pathogenesis of pyelonephritis

Meatal colonization
Ascendance of bacteria through urethra
Adherence to urothelium of the bladder
Ascendance through ureter
    (mediated by adherence, turbulence, reflux)
Adherence to urothelium of pyelocaliceal system
Pyelonephritis (promoted by high pressure, anatomical
    abnormalities, pyelotubular reflux)

After Källenius et al. (6).

a milestone in the development of our knowledge of UTIs and has greatly stimulated research in this area. The same group has shown that colonization is due to what has been called bacterial adherence to epithelial cells. This represents a specific phenomenon, which is present in some individuals and not in others and which has also been demonstrated for urothelium.

It is due to Källenius and Svenson (6) and Domingue and co-workers (7) that, in the meantime, an explanation on a bacteriological and molecular basis has been offered for the phenomenon of adherence. Adherence, at least for certain *Escherichia coli* strains, seems to be mediated by the presence of P-fimbriae and specific receptors for their protein in the epithelial cells of the urinary tract. Adherence can be interfered with in a specific way by certain glycosphingolipids. A new model for the pathogenesis of lower and higher UTIs has resulted and is summarized in Table 4. Meatal colonization occurs and is mediated by specific receptor proteins for P-fimbriae of the epithelial cells around the external meatus of the urethra. Ascendance of bacteria through the urethra occurs and may be promoted by the shortness of the female urethra and the mechanics of sexual intercourse. Elimination of the bacterial flora from the bladder by urinary flow is prevented through adhesion of the bacteria to the epithelial cells, based on specific binding of P-fimbriae. Retention of urine in the bladder may be a promoting factor. Bacteria may, or may not, then cause symptoms of cystitis, urethritis or prostatitis. Ascendance through the ureter is necessary for colonization of the upper urinary tract and for the pathogenesis of pyelonephritis. This may be promoted by reflux or stasis of urine in the upper tract due to stenosis of the ureters. Adherence to the urothelium of the pyelocaliceal system occurs, and pyelonephritis may be promoted by high pressure, anatomical changes or pyelotubular back-flow. In a careful clinical study, Domingue and co-workers (7) established that non-obstructive pyelonephritis and pyelonephritis not associated with reflux are exclusively caused by *E. coli* with P-fimbriae. Other types of bacteria, including non-P-fimbriated *E. coli*, can be the causative organisms of pyelonephritis associated with obstruction or other urological abnormalities.

Our knowledge about the other risk factors summarized in Table 3 is incomplete. The higher incidence of UTIs in younger children may be due to the relatively high incidence of urological abnormalities. The decrease with age may be associated with a decrease in severity of these abnormalities with age. For example, reflux may disappear spontaneously with age. The higher incidence of UTIs in pregnancy is poorly understood, but may be due to stasis. Asymptomatic bacteriuria during pregnancy should be treated, because the incidence of symptoms is very much higher than in the general population.

Urological abnormalities associated with recurrent UTIs are: obstruction of the upper and lower urinary tract, reflux, stones and other foreign bodies, trauma, enterovesical or vaginovesical fistulas, medullary sponge kidneys, urethral or vesical diverticula, caliceal diverticula, papillary necrosis due to diabetes mellitus or a large dose of phenacetin, and others.

Damage by UTI occurs mainly by renal damage through pyelonephritis. This can be identified by changes on X-ray studies, such as clubbing of calices and renal scarring, or by measurable loss of renal function. Pyelonephritis accounts for about 25% of end-stage renal disease, necessitating transplantation or haemodialysis. Huland and Busch (8) have shown, in a population of 42 such patients, that all of these had complicating factors mediating UTIs. In another study (9), the same authors have shown, by observation of 213 patients with recurrent UTIs during a period of 3 years, that renal scarring rarely occurs in the absence of reflux, that the incidence of new renal scarring during the observation period was 11·5% and that surgery for reflux did not change the incidence of pyelonephritic scarring. These findings may indicate that the natural history of pyelonephritis is determined by the presence of urological abnormalities on one hand but that, on the other hand, once pyelonephritis exists, the correction of the urological abnormalities may not be an important factor in the further management. The study also indicated that most renal damage occurs prior to adulthood.

When should one investigate the urinary tract in UTI? Some of the indications are summarized in Table 5; possibly the pregnant woman should be added to this list. However, the technical possibilities for a study of the urinary tract in this state are limited to the use of ultrasound and bacterial culture techniques.

Table 5

When to investigate the urinary tract in UTI

Occurrence of UTI in a child
Occurrence of UTI in a male
More than one recurrence in a woman
Failure of treatment

Treatment

Obviously, the goals of treatment should be eradication of the UTI and prevention of recurrence. The high rates of recurrence of UTIs, complicated or uncomplicated, as reported by Kunin (3) and others, remain discouraging. It is obvious, however, that factors other than antibacterial treatment are responsible for this phenomenon. In considering all the limitations of present antibacterial treatment, the first important point is that antibacterial drugs used in patients with UTIs should be specific for the urinary tract. High levels of the drug in the urine and, in the case of pyelonephritis, also in the renal tissue, should be achieved. Since the large bowel is the reservoir for bacteria causing UTI, drugs that do not induce resistance of the large bowel flora are to be preferred. The second desirable property, especially considering the possibility of long-term treatment in children, is that drugs used for treatment of UTI do not tend to induce resistance of the involved bacteria. In addition, the drugs in use ought to have a wide applicability due to a broad spectrum, lack of resistance and few side-effects. Drugs should also be efficacious and safe.

With all these requirements in mind, it is felt that the ideal management of UTIs has not yet been found. It is possible that, in the future, means of interfering with bacterial adherence will offer better treatment than antibacterial agents. For the time being, nitrofurantoins certainly qualify, among others, for the optimal treatment of UTIs.

References

(1) Kass EH. Asymptomatic infections of the urinary tract. *Trans Ass Amer Physicians* 1956; **69**: 56–74.

(2) Haag I. Een Prospectief Onderzoek naar het Beloop van Asymptomatische Bacteriurie bij Kinderen. Rotterdam: University of Rotterdam, 1977. Doctoral Thesis.

(3) Kunin CM. The natural history of recurrent bacteriuria in schoolgirls. *N Engl J Med* 1970; **282**: 1443–1448.

(4) Valkenburg HH. The epidemiology of urinary tract infections. *J Drug Ther Res* 1986; (in press).

(5) Stamey TA, Sexton CC. The role of vaginal colonization with enterobacteriaceae in recurrent urinary infections. *J Urol* 1975; **113**: 214–218.

(6) Källenius G, Svenson SB, Hultberg H, *et al*. P-fimbriae of pyelonephritogenic *Escherichia coli*: Significance for reflux and renal scarring — a hypothesis. *Infection* 1983; **11**: 73–76.

(7) Domingue GJ, Roberts HA, Laucirica R, *et al*. Pathogenic significance of P-fimbriated *Escherichia coli* in urinary tract infections. *J Urol* 1985; **133**: 983–989.

(8) Huland H, Busch R. Chronic pyelonephritis as a cause of end stage renal disease. *J Urol* 1982; **127**: 642–643.

(9) Huland H, Busch R. Pyelonephritic scarring in 213 patients with upper and lower urinary tract infections: Long-term follow up. *J Urol* 1984; **132**: 936–939.

Drug therapy and urinary tract infections: biodistribution and clinical activity of nitrofurantoin macrocrystals

J. N. CORRIERE Jr

Division of Urology, Department of Surgery,
The University of Texas Medical School
at Houston, Houston, Texas, USA

Before one can select any antibiotic to treat an infection in the urinary tract, it is essential to understand what happens to bacteria once they enter the bladder and, eventually, the kidney.

If a suspension of particles the size of bacteria, or bacteria themselves, is placed into the bladders of freely refluxing animals or humans, it will quickly ascend to the renal pelvis. However, unlike fluid reflux, which quickly returns to the bladder in a system with normal peristalsis, the particles (bacteria) can be found in the renal pelvis for up to 5 h. Moreover, these particles will enter the renal interstitial tissue of the kidney and eventually the renal lymph and blood (1,2,3,4).

Indeed, although 80–87% of refluxed bacteria eventually leaves the renal pelvis by way of the ureter, the rest appears to exit by way of the renal lymph and blood. In the normal upper tract, it takes up to 10 min for blood stream egress to occur, but, in the presence of a ligated ureter or in the pyelonephritic organ, bacteria can be found in the renal vein blood within 2–2·5 min of renal inoculation (2). Bacteria also enter the renal lymphatics in both the normal and obstructed upper urinary tracts fairly freely but pyelonephritis seems to seal the lymphatics and prohibits the exit of particles and bacteria by this route.

Since lymph fluid represents a derivative of interstitial fluid, analysis of antibiotic concentrations in renal lymph can be a method of defining antibiotic concentrations in the interstitial fluid of the kidney (5). Another way to evaluate renal tissue distribution of antibiotics is the use of autoradiographs (6).

Unfortunately, these techniques will only identify lymph or tissue concentrations of the drug or radioactivity, which may represent microbiologically active or inactive drug metabolites. Recently we investigated the *in vivo* distribution of nitrofurantoin macrocrystals* in the human and a subhuman primate system and directly assessed

*Nitrofurantoin macrocrystals, originated by Norwich Eaton Pharmaceuticals, Inc., is distributed under the following registered trade marks: Benelux, Furadantine MC®; West Germany, Furadantin Retard®; USA, Canada and UK, Macrodantin®; France, Furadantine®; Latin America, Macrodantina®.

Recent advances in the treatment of urinary tract infections, edited by F. H. Schröder, 1985: Royal Society of Medicine Services International Congress and Symposium Series No. 97, published by Royal Society of Medicine Services Limited.

the bactericidal activity of the drug concentrated in the human kidney on known urinary tract pathogens (7).

Autoradiographic drug distribution

Four female squirrel monkeys received an oral dose of ^{14}C nitrofurantoin macro-crystals ($8\cdot8$ mg/kg). Then $0\cdot5$, 1, 2 or 3 h later they were sacrificed and whole body radioautography was performed as described previously (8). One animal was given a placebo and analysed as a control. Blood and urine samples were collected at the time of sacrifice and analysed for nitrofurantoin content (9).

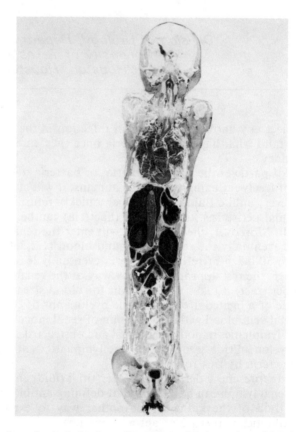

Figure 1. Composite of whole body radioautograph of monkey 3 h after administration of oral nitrofurantoin macrocrystals. Note wide distribution to all tissues except brain and spinal cord. (After Boileau et al. (7), reproduced with permission of J Urol.)

Nitrofurantoin macrocrystals is seen to be rapidly absorbed and distributed to all tissues and organs except the central nervous system (Fig. 1). Highest drug concentrations were in the liver, gastrointestinal tract, kidney, bladder epithelium and urine (Figs 2 and 3). Peak blood and urine levels were seen 2 h after dosing (Table 1). Urinary levels of the drug were equal to levels in the renal parenchyma and renal pelvis.

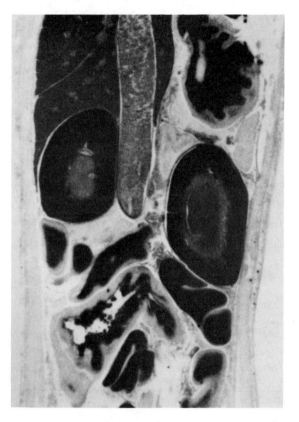

Figure 2. Close-up of abdominal organ distributions of nitrofurantoin macrocrystals. Heaviest concentrations are in the kidney, liver and gastrointestinal tract. (After Boileau et al. (7), reproduced with permission of J Urol.)

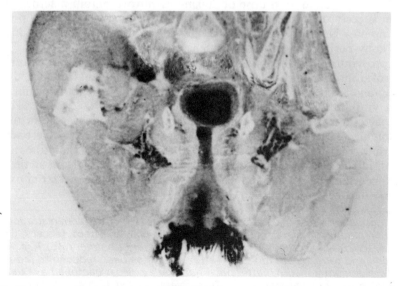

Figure 3. Close-up of pelvic organs. High bladder and urine concentrations are evident. (After Boileau et al. (7), reproduced with permission of J Urol.)

Table 1

Concentrations of nitrofurantoin in urine and plasma after an 8·8 mg/kg oral dose in the squirrel monkey

Time after dose (h)	Plasma (μg/ml)	Urine (μg/ml)	Urine/plasma concentration ratio
0·5	0·31	0·80	2·58
1·0	2·22	7·50	3·38
2·0	3·83	11·80	3·10
3·0	1·85	8·99	4·86

After Boileau *et al.* (7), reproduced with permission of *J Urol.*

Table 2

Strains of organisms susceptible to nitrofurantoin macrocrystals

Pathogen	Strain
E. coli	Clinical isolate
Proteus mirabilis	WT 844
Staph. epidermidis	9492
Staph. epidermidis	TSB 9609
Proteus	WT 67C
Klebsiella pneumoniae	9398
Klebsiella oxytoca	SPT 9262
Staph. saprophyticum	ST 2409
Strept. faecalis	WT 2390

After Boileau *et al.* (7), reproduced with permission of *J Urol.*

Bioautography

Five patients received an oral dose of 200 mg of nitrofurantoin macrocrystals and five patients received a placebo 24 h and 2 h before a nephrectomy for a polar renal cell carcinoma. Normal tissue was removed from the excised kidneys and bioautography performed on the specimens (10).

In this procedure, thin slices of tissue are inoculated with an 18-h culture of one of the nitrofurantoin-susceptible bacteria isolated from human urine listed in Table 2. The sections are then overlaid with a solution of triphenyltetrazoleum chloride immediately, 6 and 12 h after the bacterial inoculation.

Living bacteria on the tissue suspension will reduce the colourless tetrazoleum salt to an insoluble red dye. Therefore, red-coloured tissue means viable bacteria are present, while colourless areas contain dead bacteria. This test, therefore, is a visual correlate of nitrofurantoin's bactericidal activity. As shown in Fig. 4, all the bacteria tested reduced the dye applied immediately, but by 12 h after bacterial overlay all the bacteria had been killed.

Figure 4 (opposite). Human kidney tissue removed 2 h after administration of oral nitrofurantoin macrocrystals. Bacteria inoculum: (I) E. coli, (II) Strept. faecalis, (III) Staph. epidermidis, (IV) Staph. saprophyticum. (A) Tissue before treatment. (B) Tissue overlaid with bacteria and tetrazoleum mixture. Tetrazoleum has been reduced to red formazan dye. (C) Tetrazoleum added 6 h after bacterial overlay. Most bacteria have been killed, little tetrazoleum has been reduced. (D) Tetrazoleum added 12 h after bacterial overlay. All bacteria have been killed. Tissue remains as colourless as before treatment. After Boileau et al. (7), reproduced with permission of J Urol.)

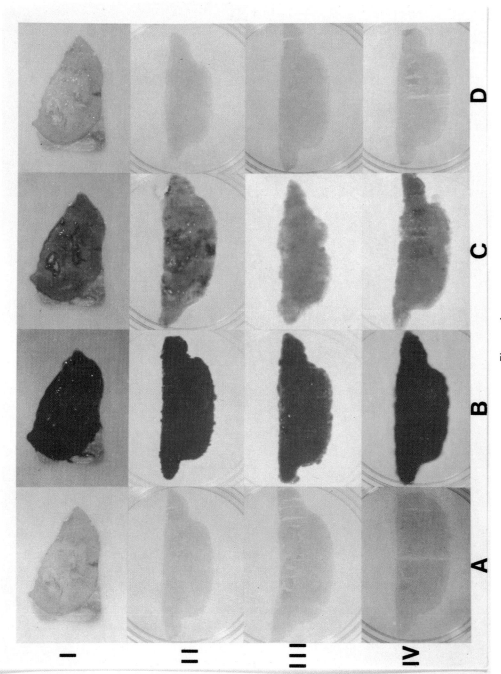

Figure 4

Discussion

When one is choosing drug therapy for urinary tract infection (UTI), there are a number of considerations which should be borne in mind. Of importance are: host factors (e.g. hypersensitivity reaction to a particular drug; structural defects of the urinary tract); urinary tract specificity of the drug; bacterial resistance to therapy, and safety of therapy. This paper deals with aspects of one of these factors: the biodistribution of the drug and, thus, urinary tract specificity and clinical activity.

Looking at the pharmacokinetics of a compound administered orally for use in the treatment of UTI, one would ideally want the following properties: (a) rapid absorption and (b) urinary tract specificity. Rapid and complete absorption of the drug from the gut means that there is little or no residual drug to reach and alter the normal bowel flora. Any active drug which reaches the faecal reservoir can rapidly select for resistance among the micro-organisms which occasionally or habitually infect the perineum.

One would also want a compound with a distribution and excretion profile such that the drug is chiefly concentrated in the urinary tract, which, obviously, is where the clinical activity is desired. The other side of this coin—a low serum drug concentration—is a positive advantage in UTI therapy, since the aim is to attain an adequate bactericidal drug concentration in the urinary tract without affecting the ecological balance of the normal flora at any other point in the body. If the serum levels of a drug in the body reach antibacterial significance, then bowel and vaginal flora can be altered. For example, a significant effect on the vaginal flora is seen with oral preparations of the tetracyclines and penicillins, and the trimethoprim/ sulphamethoxazole combination is known to attain a serum level which can significantly affect the bowel flora.

The drug of choice in many instances of UTI is the macrocrystalline form of nitrofurantoin. (This form is preferred since the generic compound, nitrofurantoin, has marked gastrointestinal side-effects and patient compliance is poor.) Nitrofurantoin macrocrystals is rapidly and completely absorbed, having a low, non-bactericidal serum concentration and a short half-life of 19 min. (Owing to this rapid half-life, however, nitrofurantoin compounds should be avoided in patients with impaired renal function.) The urinary tract is the only site at which the drug is present in bactericidal concentrations. It is distributed in the urine, medullary tubular lumen, interstitial space and renal lymph. Conklin and Hailey (11) found that the mean urinary drug recoveries in man following orally administered nitrofurantoin macrocrystals were 35–37·9%, with urinary concentrations well in excess of that required to kill the majority of urinary tract infecting organisms.

The urinary tract specificity of nitrofurantoin macrocrystals may be the reason why this compound has shown no selection and no altered resistance profile in the 30 years or so since it first became available for use.

Summary

Since bacterial infection in the kidney is centred in the interstitial tissue, a drug that allows a high interstitial fluid concentration should be employed to treat pyelonephritis adequately. The urine concentrations and renal lymph concentrations both reflect the level of the drug in the renal parenchyma (12). Whether it is the tissue level or the urine level of nitrofurantoin that actually kills the bacteria is not important from a clinical viewpoint.

The present report gives direct evidence of the intrarenal distribution of the drug, as well as proving that nitrofurantoin macrocrystals is a true bactericidal agent for known urinary pathogens in the interstitium of the human kidney, and qualifying it as an ideal drug for the treatment of UTIs.

References

(1) Corriere JN Jr, Lipschultz LI, Judson FN, *et al*. Autoradiographic localization of refluxed live and dead *Escherichia coli* and sulfur colloid particles in the rat kidney. *Invest Urol* 1969; **6**: 364.

(2) Corriere JN Jr, Lipschultz LI, Judson FN, *et al*. The use of 99 mTc labeled sulfur colloid to study particle dynamics in the urinary tract. II. Routes of removal from the renal pelvis in normal and pyelonephritic kidney. *J Urol* 1970; **103**: 393.

(3) Corriere JN Jr, Murphy JJ. Vesicoureteral reflux and the intrarenal lymphatic system in the rat. *Invest Urol* 1967; **4**: 556.

(4) Corriere JN Jr, Lipschultz LI. The clearance of refluxed bacteria-sized sulfur colloid particles from the human kidney. In: Skinner DB, Ebert PA, eds. *Current topics in surgical research*. New York: Academic Press, Inc., 1971; Vol. 3, 191–196.

(5) Cockett ATK, Roberts AP, Moore R. Significance of antibacterial levels in the renal lymph during treatment for pyelonephritis. *J Urol* 1966; **95**: 164.

(6) Currie GA, Little PJ, McDonald SJ. The localization of cephaloridine and nitrofurantoin in the kidney. *Nephron* 1966; **3**: 282.

(7) Boileau MA, Corriere JN Jr, Liss RH. Visualization of bactericidal concentrations of nitrofurantoin macrocrystals in primate and human urinary tract tissue. *J Urol* 1983; **130**: 1010.

(8) Liss RH, Letourneau RJ, Schepis JP. Distribution of ethambutal in primate tissues and cells. *Am Rev Respir Dis* 1981; **123**: 529.

(9) Liss RH, Kensler CJ. Radioautographic methods for physiologic disposition and toxicology studies. In: Mehlman, Shapiro, Blumenthal, eds. *Advances in modern toxicology. New concepts in safety evaluation*. New York: Wiley, 1976; 273–305.

(10) Tubaro E, Bulgini MJ. Cytotoxic and antifungal agents: their body distribution and tissue affinity. *Nature* 1968; **218**: 395.

(11) Conklin JD, Hailey FJ. Urinary drug excretion in man during oral dosage of different nitrofurantoin formulations. *Clin Pharmacol Ther* 1969; **10**: 534.

(12) Stamey TA, Fair WR, Timothy MM, *et al*. Serum versus urinary antimicrobial concentrations in cure of urinary tract infections. *N Engl J Med* 1974; **291**: 1159.

Development of bacterial resistance during the treatment of urinary tract infections: a constant clinical challenge

W. BRUMFITT and J. M. T. HAMILTON-MILLER

Urinary Infection Clinic and Department of Medical Microbiology, Royal Free Hospital and School of Medicine, London, UK

For a proper understanding of bacterial drug resistance and its implications, it is necessary to appreciate that history has shown that acquisition of resistance to antibiotics appears inevitable. There are variations in the rate and extent to which such acquisition takes place, but sooner or later, as a consequence of the genetic and biochemical versatility of bacteria, it will occur.

Experience gained over the period of about 50 years which has so far made up the 'antibiotic era' gives us ideas about how best to combat resistance, in terms of reducing its advance on the one hand, and, on the other, of designing new compounds that will be active against bacteria which have acquired resistance to existing antibacterials. We have been able to identify antibacterial agents to which resistance is easily acquired (nalidixic acid) or acquired only with difficulty (nitrofurantoin) and which bacterial species acquire resistance readily (*Pseudomonas aeruginosa, Staphylococcus epidermidis*) or with difficulty (*Streptococcus pyogenes* Group A).

It is of the greatest practical importance that clinicians know which antibiotics are likely to be the most effective in a certain set of circumstances, so that treatment of life-threatening infections can commence before formal sensitivity tests have been carried out ('best-guess treatment'). For this reason, continuous monitoring of sensitivity patterns is an important part of the overall study of the emergence of bacterial resistance.

Resistance transfer and mechanisms

Before discussing in detail problems associated with bacterial resistance with reference to the treatment of urinary infections, it is essential to recapitulate some points concerning resistance in general.

Recent advances in the treatment of urinary tract infections, edited by F. H. Schröder, 1985: Royal Society of Medicine Services International Congress and Symposium Series No. 97, published by Royal Society of Medicine Services Limited.

Resistance arises in a bacterial cell owing to a change in the DNA. This can come about either by spontaneous mutation or by the acquisition, from another organism, of the gene specifying drug resistance. It should be stressed that this genetic change must be followed by selection of the resistant individuals if resistance is to be of clinical significance. Antibiotic use kills sensitive organisms and allows only the more resistant bacteria to survive, a phenomenon referred to as selection pressure.

Spontaneous mutations

The rate at which spontaneous mutation occurs is a characteristic both of the type of bacterium and of the drug under consideration. For many of the drugs used for the treatment of urinary infection, the rate of spontaneous mutation to resistance is too low to be of significance (namely $< 1:10^{10}$). However, examples of antibiotics that are affected in this respect are nalidixic acid, streptomycin and rifampicin. For Gram-negative bacteria the incidence of spontaneously resistant mutants is between $1:10^6$ and $1:10^8$ for these compounds. It is thus clear that if a significant bacteriuria of 10^5 organisms per ml persists for 1 day (during which at least 1 litre of urine is passed), sufficient bacteria will have been present in the urinary tract long enough for there to be an excellent statistical chance that at least one resistant mutant will have been present. Such resistance is chromosomal, of relatively high level, occurs in a single step and is permanent. In the case of rifampicin, resistance is due to an altered DNA-directed RNA polymerase, for nalidixic acid an altered gyrase α-subunit and for streptomycin an altered protein (S12) on the 30S ribosome, each of which is insusceptible to inhibition by the respective antibiotic.

This type of resistance is avoided in the clinical situation by the use of antibiotic combinations (such as rifampicin plus trimethoprim) or in the case of nalidixic acid by administering the drug at frequent intervals (6-hourly) in order to maintain adequate urinary concentrations which will avoid the emergence of resistant mutants. Another approach would be to choose an antimicrobial agent such as nitrofurantoin, which rarely develops resistance in the clinical setting.

It should be noted that emergence of resistance does not always occur when these antibiotics are used. Resistant bacteria emerge in only about 30% of patients treated with rifampicin alone (1). Provided high enough doses are used for short periods, streptomycin has been shown to be very effective therapy for urinary infections (2), owing to its extremely rapid rate of killing. Aminoglycosides other than streptomycin bind to more than one ribosomal protein, and so not only does single-step mutation to high level resistance to compounds such as gentamicin and kanamycin not occur, but also there is no cross-resistance between streptomycin and other aminoglycosides. Similarly, other members of the quinolone family (e.g. cinoxacin, norfloxacin and ciprofloxacin) do not seem to select for resistance as rapidly as does nalidixic acid, but experience with these compounds is still quite limited.

A multi-step pattern of chromosomal resistance has been occurring among gonococci for the past 40 years, but this has not been observed by us in organisms causing urinary infections.

Transferable resistance

Exchange of DNA between bacteria can transfer resistance: this process can be shown to occur with chromosomal DNA by transformation, transduction or conjugation (3).

However, none of these phenomena has been shown to be important in the spread of bacterial drug resistance under clinical circumstances. On the other hand, extra-chromosomal DNA (plasmids or R-factors) is of prime importance: in both Gram-negative and Gram-positive bacteria, plasmids are transferred by conjugation (although the precise mechanisms appear to be different). Plasmids may carry determinants for resistance to many antibiotics simultaneously: transfer of these gives rise to multiple resistance. It should be noted that plasmids are relatively unstable entities and in the absence of a continuous selection pressure are lost at a relatively high rate. Plasmid-mediated resistance thus tends to disappear if antibiotics are not being used. However, those plasmids that are capable of integration into the chromosome ('transposons') are stable while in the integrated state.

Practical aspects of resistance: clinical and laboratory

As has been discussed above, any use of antibiotics (whether rational or irrational) selects for resistance. It is important to distinguish whether the strains that emerge are those with acquired resistance (e.g. due to an R-factor) or those with intrinsic resistance. The latter situation is often referred to as 'super-infection' and is a characteristic feature of the use of certain broad-spectrum antibiotics. For example, the use of a number of cephalosporins such as latamoxef (Moxalactam®) may be followed by infection with *Strept. faecalis*, an organism which is intrinsically resistant to cephalosporins. Similarly, when aztreonam was used to treat pneumonias caused by Gram-negative organisms, *Strept. pneumoniae* infections followed in about one-third of the patients (4). In our experience neither of these situations is a common one in urinary infections, although both occur from time to time in individual patients.

Since 1973 we have held a Urinary Infection Clinic at the Royal Free Hospital, with physicians from the Department of Medical Microbiology seeing the patients, allocating treatment and carrying out follow-up. Detailed records, both clinical and microbiological, are kept. Those patients who satisfy criteria laid down in strict protocols are entered into studies. Within the specific protocols of these studies, 607 patients have been treated for acute infections, and long-term antimicrobial prophylaxis (1-year treatment) has been prescribed for 345. Analysing the results of such treatments over the period of 13 years has afforded an invaluable and probably unique insight into changing patterns of resistance in a specific population. During the same time we have also analysed resistance in organisms isolated from urinary infections occurring in other populations.

Resistance in strains isolated from patients suffering from recurrent urinary infections

These are results obtained from patients attending our Urinary Infection Clinic. Such patients are heavily exposed to antibiotics, as they may suffer from 12 (or occasionally even more) symptomatic attacks per year, for which they have previously been given a course of antibiotic treatment by their family doctor. Treatment for acute lower tract infections is usually a 5–10 day course of co-trimoxazole or amoxycillin (amoxicillin). Thus it is reasonable to assume that resistant organisms are more likely to occur in these patients than in almost any other group. As *Escherichia coli* is much the most common species that causes urinary infections (in general practice 80–90%),

Table 1

Sensitivity of bacteria isolated from patients with recurrent infections attending Urinary Infection Clinic at Royal Free Hospital, analysed on a year-to-year basis

		Infecting organisms sensitive to indicated antibiotics (%)								
		Cephradine		Nitrofurantoin		Trimethoprim		Ampicillin		Sulphonamide
Study no.	Duration of study	E. coli	Overall	E. coli	Overall	E. coli	Overall	E. coli	Overall	E. coli	Overall
1	1975–77	100	98	98	88	94	92	89	89	70	76
2	1977–80	100	100	100	98	92	88	75	77	69	70
3	1978–79	100	86	98	84	95	88	82	78	58	52
4	1978–80	97	93	100	98	95	89	90	88	79	76
5	1979–81	97	89	100	95	97	93	84	88	67	69
6	1981–82	95	91	100	96	71	69	71	70	61	66
7	1982–84	96	95	100	97	76	79	68	68	58	61

(Data from references 5, 6, 7, 8, 9, 10 and 11).

we have concentrated our attention on this species in our analyses of resistance to ampicillin, cephradine, nitrofurantoin, sulphonamide and trimethoprim. This has been carried out continuously over the past 10 years on strains of *E. coli* causing acute infections.

Our results (Table 1) indicate that there has been a steady fall in the incidence of sensitivity to ampicillin (and amoxycillin) and to sulphonamide over the years. Resistance has been increasing at a rate of roughly 10% every 5 years. On the other hand, cephradine and nitrofurantoin have shown virtually no decrease in their antibacterial action.

Trimethoprim is a somewhat special case: after an initial period of years during which resistance remained at a steady and low level, the situation deteriorated from about 1979. This matter is discussed in more detail below.

Mecillinam (amdinocillin) sensitivity was monitored between 1977 and 1982 and rifampicin from 1977 to 1981. During these periods we found only two out of 254 strains of *E. coli* to be resistant to mecillinam, while all 188 strains tested against rifampicin were sensitive to this antibiotic. The high incidence of sensitivity to these antibiotics reflects the restricted use of these compounds in the UK.

More recently, with the worsening position of ampicillin (and amoxycillin), we have turned our attention to the combination of clavulanic acid plus amoxycillin (Augmentin®). During 1983 we found 63% of *E. coli* strains to be sensitive to ampicillin but 91·6% were sensitive to clavulanic acid plus amoxycillin (12). The above figures suggest it may soon no longer be a useful exercise to test urine isolates routinely against either ampicillin or sulphonamide.

We suspect that at least some of the increased incidence of resistance to trimethoprim observed in our patients (which was substantially higher than the 6% incidence found in the general population at the same time) may have been due to the fact that we were using trimethoprim as long-term prophylaxis from mid-1979 to mid-1983. Short-term (7–14 days) treatment with co-trimoxazole or with trimethoprim alone results in the total elimination of faecal coliforms followed by the reappearance of fully sensitive strains after the end of treatment (13). On the other hand, we discovered that long-term treatment (12 months) with trimethoprim, in a dose of 100 mg daily, resulted in the emergence of trimethoprim-resistant *E. coli* in the faeces (16). A detailed study of flora from monthly rectal swabs taken from patients on a 12-month course of trimethoprim showed that about 5% of patients acquired trimethoprim-resistant *E. coli* during each month of treatment.

Since the middle of 1983 our choice of long-term prophylactic treatment has been either cephradine, nitrofurantoin macrocrystals* or norfloxacin. (The latter antibiotic is not yet generally available in Great Britain.) We are at present not using long-term trimethoprim in the Urinary Infection Clinic. It will therefore be very interesting to see whether the incidence of trimethoprim resistance in this population shows a progressive fall. The answer to this intriguing question should soon be answered as a result of continuous monitoring of our patients.

It was a very striking finding that not only was there no acquisition of resistance to nitrofurantoin macrocrystals during long-term treatment but also that intrinsically resistant organisms, such as *Proteus* spp. or *Ps. aeruginosa*, were not selected in the faecal flora (15,16). The result of this combination of events was that break-through infection was a rare event in patients taking nitrofurantoin macrocrystals.

---

*Nitrofurantoin macrocrystals, originated by Norwich Eaton Pharmaceuticals, Inc., is distributed under the following registered trade marks: Benelux, Furadantine MC®; West Germany, Furadantin Retard®; USA, Canada and UK, Macrodantin®; France, Furadantine®; Latin America, Macrodantina®.

Table 2

Changes in resistance to trimethoprim in different bacterial species over various periods

Incidence of resistance to trimethoprim at different times

Bacterial species	1973–1975	1979		1981		1985	
		GP	Hospital	GP	Hospital	GP	Hospital
E. coli	1·4%	4·1%	7·7%	6·2%	9·0%	20·0%	19·5%
K. pneumoniae	18·3%	27·0%	21·4%	11·8%	16·1%	18·0%	20·0%
Pr. mirabilis	2·1%	3·0%	21·3%	15·8%	14·3%	34·0%	30·0%
Enterobacter spp.	12·0%	13·9%		16·7%		27%	
All isolates (no. of strains tested)	3·2% (4168)	15·5% (5462)		6% (744)	13·0% (1956)	21·6% (499)	25·8% (662)
				11% overall		24% overall	

(Data from references 17, 18, 19 and 24 (and authors' unpublished work).)

Resistance in strains isolated from general practice and hospital patients

Trimethoprim

Since 1973 we have been monitoring resistance to trimethoprim among bacteria causing urinary infection. During this time it has become apparent that it is essential to survey isolates continuously for at least 3 months as otherwise there is a danger that the figures obtained may be unrepresentative, owing to the fact that there may be wide variations from month to month (17).

Our results are shown in Table 2. Several interesting facts emerge from a consideration of those data. There was an increase in the incidence of resistance between 1973/5 and 1979 of about four-fold overall, which was most marked for *E. coli* and *Proteus mirabilis*. Two years later the situation was virtually unchanged but by 1985 we had observed another increase: an approximate doubling in overall resistance to a figure of 24%. By contrast, the incidence of resistance in *Klebsiella pneumoniae* strains does not seem to have increased over the past 10 years.

Another striking and unexpected finding is that the incidence of bacterial resistance is now virtually the same in hospital patients and in patients living at home, whereas in previous years it was higher in hospital isolates. This finding was puzzling at first sight, as it would be expected that the absence of selection pressure outside the hospital environment would result in a loss of R-factors (the usual vectors of most antibiotic resistance). Under these circumstances, therefore, a lower incidence of resistance in non-hospital isolates would be predicted since exposure to trimethoprim would be low. However, the apparent anomaly is explicable if resistance to trimethoprim is now mainly carried on a transposon: the genes responsible for resistance hence become chromosomal and thus stable. The change observed is presumably due to transposons such as Tn7 becoming more widely distributed as time has passed.

Other antibiotics

We have also carried out slightly less detailed but nevertheless comprehensive surveys of sensitivity patterns to several commonly used antibiotics in bacteria isolated from urines of both hospital and general practice patients. Results are shown in Table 3. It is again clear that cephradine and nitrofurantoin are more likely to be active than other antimicrobials, both against *E. coli* and against all isolates studied. In isolates from general practice patients there is now little to choose between the overall activity of ampicillin, trimethoprim and sulphonamide, all being active against 65–80% of strains tested. Hospital isolates are only slightly less susceptible than those from patients living at home.

The impact of acquired bacterial resistance on clinical results

We have recently experienced two striking examples of how important acquired resistance may be in affecting strategy and results of treatment of patients.

Table 3

Resistance to five antibiotics among urinary isolates from hospital and domiciliary patients in different years

Strains sensitive (%)[a]

	Cephradine		Nitrofurantoin		Ampicillin		Trimethoprim		Sulphonamide	
	E. coli	All	E. coli	All	E. coli	All	E. coli	All	E. coli	All
June 1984: Hospital	98 (116)	78 (200)	99	85	60	63	74	71	53	53
August 1983: GP	96 (149)	89 (210)	96	90	72	80	89	88	67	70
January 1984: GP	97 (208)	90 (294)	96	92	74	77	89	87	68	69
1985: GP	95 (350)	90 (499)	96	90	66	70	80	78	62	65
Hospital	95 (377)	82 (662)	95	87	61	68	80	74	62	62

[a]No. of strains investigated in parentheses.

The first example was that the unexpected increase in resistance to trimethoprim altered the way in which we carried out a study comparing co-trimoxazole with clavulanic acid plus amoxycillin (8). We were forced to abandon the original protocol, by which patients were entered only if their infecting organism was sensitive to both study drugs, because so many strains were found to be trimethoprim resistant. Instead we adopted a modified, more flexible approach to treatment, obtaining results that we feel are more relevant to the practising clinician than are those obtained by more conventional trials of the type favoured by regulatory authorities. This trial and its implications are fully discussed elsewhere (8,20).

The second example is even more striking. It is given by the results of a comparative trial of long-term prophylaxis using nitrofurantoin macrocrystals or trimethoprim, each at a dose of 100 mg at night for 12 months. During the course of this study (as pointed out in a previous section), it was observed that, in patients taking trimethoprim, resistance to trimethoprim emerged in faecal coliforms as well as in the bacteria colonizing the periurethral area. As a result of this, many breakthrough infections were observed in those patients with trimethoprim-resistant strains. Consequently, the therapeutic value of trimethoprim was seriously diminished. By contrast, no emergence of resistance to nitrofurantoin was observed (either in faecal or in periurethral flora), and no breakthrough infections by resistant strains occurred in the group of patients taking nitrofurantoin macrocrystals.

This trial showed conclusively that treatment with nitrofurantoin macrocrystals was therapeutically significantly more effective than trimethoprim in preventing both dysuria and frequency as well as bacteriuria. This difference can be explained solely by the fact that resistance emerged in those patients treated with trimethoprim but did not occur in the patients treated with nitrofurantoin macrocrystals. The major difficulty encountered with nitrofurantoin macrocrystals was that a number of patients had to abandon treatment owing to the onset of nausea. Interestingly, this most often occurred during the first month of long-term treatment, which suggests that some patients are unduly susceptible to this side-effect. In addition, taking nitrofurantoin macrocrystals with food or milk may lessen the incidence of nausea.

Ways to minimize risk of resistance emerging

As stated above, it is the amount of antibiotic use that can often explain the emergence of resistance. Contrary to popular belief, and with few exceptions, it is unusual for bacteria infecting the urinary tract to become resistant to the therapeutic agent being used for treatment. We believe that selection takes place in the gut, and the resistant bacteria subsequently spread to the periurethral area and initiate infection by ascending the urethra. It is therefore appropriate to consider the effect of antibiotics on the gut flora when attempting to prevent the emergence of resistance. Some antibiotics rapidly select resistant coliforms in the gut; ampicillin and tetracycline being examples (21). Carriage may be maintained for long periods of time after antibiotic treatment has ended (22). Furthermore, the administration of one antibiotic (such as tetracycline) may cause resistance to several other antibiotics (21). The explanation for this apparently paradoxical phenomenon is that several determinants of resistance are often carried on a single R-factor. The main reason for selection of resistance in the gut flora is incomplete absorption of antibiotic following oral administration, so that bacteria in the large intestine are exposed to the antibiotic.

Acute infections

The use of antibiotics for acute infections should therefore be restricted to cases in which their use is entirely appropriate. Thus either completely absorbed compounds like cephalexin or cephradine should be used, so that the antibiotic does not reach the bowel flora, or, alternatively, compounds to which resistance only rarely emerges should be used. Nitrofurantoin macrocrystals is effective in both categories, in that the compound is completely absorbed in the upper gastrointestinal tract *and* resistance seldom occurs.

Courses of treatment should be as short as is compatible with an optimal cure rate. There is no evidence that any benefit accrues by extending the period of treatment of an acute urinary infection beyond 7 days. Also, because antibiotic is concentrated in the urine it is easy to exceed the optimal dose. For example, on the data sheet (23) the dose of cephradine recommended for urinary infection is greater than that for respiratory tract infection. This is in spite of the published data showing that urinary levels of cephradine are very much higher than those in the blood.

Long-term treatment

When long-term antimicrobial prophylaxis is considered necessary it is essential to use an appropriate compound. As will be clear from the above, sulphonamide and ampicillin are unsuitable, as resistance in the bowel flora will soon emerge and breakthrough infections will be likely to occur with resistant organisms even though the bladder urine contains antibiotic. At the present time trimethoprim may be effective for several months but, as we have shown (14,16), if resistant gut flora appear then breakthrough infections with trimethoprim-resistant organisms are, sooner or later, an inevitable consequence. Antiseptics such as methenamine salts do not select for resistance but they are not as effective clinically as are nitrofurantoin macrocrystals or cephradine (15; and authors' unpublished observations).

The newer quinolones such as norfloxacin are, at present, being investigated. These do not appear to give rise to resistant variants in the gut, despite the fact that they are poorly absorbed after oral administration; for instance, both ciprofloxacin and norfloxacin are found in concentrations of 1 mg/g or greater in the faeces (25,26). Furthermore, the newer quinolones investigated by us do not allow overgrowth by intrinsically resistant species. However, these new derivatives related to nalidixic acid have only been studied for a relatively short period of time and comparative clinical trials will be needed to establish their place in long-term prophylaxis of urinary tract infections. Preliminary results with norfloxacin are extremely encouraging (Brumfitt *et al.*, unpublished) but doubts about toxicity of some quinolones have resulted in caution in the use of these compounds in Britain.

Variation among antibiotics in ability to produce resistance

The question must now be asked as to why some antibiotics seem to encourage the emergence of resistant variants at a rapid rate, while others do so only slowly or not at all. Resistance to ampicillin and to sulphonamide is usually carried on an R-factor. Several surveys have shown that one particular R-factor (known as TEM) is found in about 70% of all R+ strains (27,28). This R-factor carries a determinant for the production of TEM β-lactamase—which rapidly destroys ampicillin—as well as conferring sulphonamide resistance by a separate mechanism. It is significant that cephradine and cephalexin are not hydrolysed by TEM β-lactamase. Thus, bacteria containing the TEM R-factor will be resistant to ampicillin and sulphonamide but sensitive to cephradine and cephalexin.

Nitrofurantoin has to be chemically reduced to active metabolites before it is microbiologically active: this reaction takes place within the bacterial cell and is brought about by reductases, of which at least three exist in *E. coli*. Resistance will occur if one or more of these reductases is lost by mutation. Although it has recently been reported that resistance to nitrofurantoin may be carried on an R-factor (29), nonetheless, as we have shown above (Tables 1 and 3), the overall incidence remains low. This is explicable if loss of reductases seriously impairs bacterial viability. Details of the mode of action of nitrofurans are not at present understood, except it is known that they act on nucleic acids and consequently result in cell death.

Summary

Development of resistance of an organism in the *urine* to a specific antimicrobial agent is unusual with most of the commonly used antimicrobial agents. However, resistance can emerge in the *bowel* even during very short-term treatment (e.g. 3 days) with agents such as amoxycillin. Such resistance may subsequently spread in the community, creating an ecological hazard. In the area served by the Royal Free Hospital, for example, about 40% of *E. coli* strains isolated from acute urinary infections are amoxycillin resistant.

Long-term therapy of 6–12 months is an effective means of preventing recurrent urinary infections in problem patients. Again, resistant bowel organisms may spread to colonize the area around the patient's urethra and cause 'breakthrough' infections. The choice of suitable agents for long-term treatment is limited but it is clear that the preferred agent will be a compound to which resistance only rarely emerges. A compound which is completely absorbed following oral administration is less likely to affect normal bowel flora, so a circular process of reinfection with resistant organisms arising from the bowel reservoir is avoided.

Our experience in the Urinary Infection Clinic at the Royal Free Hospital has illustrated this problem and has given some direction as to the selection of the most suitable therapy among existing compounds. Regarding the sensitivity of infecting organisms to the antimicrobials used in our studies, only cephradine and nitrofurantoin macrocrystals have maintained (cephradine) or improved (nitrofurantoin) their position since 1975. These figures (Table 1) reflect the properties of the antimicrobial agents: nitrofurantoin macrocrystals, for instance, being both urinary tract specific and wholly absorbed following oral administration, and not prone to the development of resistance.

References

(1) Kissling M, Bergamini N. *Chemotherapy* 1981; **27**: 368–402.
(2) Barber M, Garrod LP. *Antibiotic and chemotherapy*. London: E & S Livingstone. 1963.
(3) Bryan LF. *Antimicrobial drug resistance*. London: Academic Press, 1984.

(4) Davies BI, Maesen EPV, Teengs JP. *J Antimicrob Chemother* 1985; **15**: 375–384.

(5) Brumfitt W, Hamilton-Miller JMT. *Infection* 1982; **10**: 149–152.

(6) Brumfitt W, Hamilton-Miller JMT. *Drugs under Experimental and Clinical Research* 1981; 7: 335–344.

(7) Brumfitt W, Hamilton-Miller JMT. *Chemotherapy* 1984; **30**: 270–275.

(8) Brumfitt W, Hamilton-Miller JMT. *Br J Clin Pract* 1985; **39**: 346–351.

(9) Brumfitt W, Hamilton-Miller JMT, Ludlam H, Damjanovic V, Gargan RA. *Infection* 1982; **10**: 280–284.

(10) Brumfitt W, Smith GW, Hamilton-Miller JMT, Bax R. *J Antimicrob Chemother* 1985; (in press).

(11) Cooper J. Brumfitt W, Hamilton-Miller JMT. *J Antimicrob Chemother* 1980; **6**: 231–239.

(12) Brumfitt W, Hamilton-Miller JMT. *Lancet* 1983; **ii**: 566.

(13) Knothe H. *Chemotherapy* 1973; **18**: 285–296.

(14) Brumfitt W, Hamilton-Miller JMT, Gargan RA, Cooper J, Smith GW. *J Urol* 1983; **130**: 1110–1114.

(15) Brumfitt W, Cooper J, Hamilton-Miller JMT. *J Urol* 1981; **126**: 71–74.

(16) Brumfitt W, Smith GW, Hamilton-Miller JMT, Gargan RA. *J Antimicrob Chemother* 1985; **16**: 111–120.

(17) Hamilton-Miller JMT, Gooding A, Brumfitt W. *J Clin Pathol* 1981; **34**: 439–442.

(18) Brumfitt W, Hamilton-Miller JMT, Gooding A. *Lancet* 1980; **i**: 1409–1410.

(19) Grey D, Hamilton-Miller JMT, Brumfitt W. *Chemotherapy* 1979; **25**: 147–156.

(20) Brumfitt W, Hamilton-Miller JMT. *J Antimicrob Chemother* 1984; **13** (suppl B): 121–133.

(21) Datta N, Faiers MC, Reeves DS, Brumfitt W, Ørskov F, Ørskov I. *Lancet* 1971; **i**: 312–315.

(22) Hartley CL, Richmond MH *Br Med J* 1975; **iv**: 71–74.

(23) Association of the British Pharmaceutical Industry. *Data sheet compendium*. London: Datapharm Publications, 1985; 1473.

(24) Brumfitt W, Hamilton-Miller JMT, Wood A. *J Antimicrob Chemother* 1983; **11**: 503–509.

(25) Brumfitt W, Franklin I, Grady D, Hamilton-Miller JMT, Iliffe A. *Antimicrob Agents Chemother* 1984; **26**: 757–761.

(26) Cofsky RD, du Bouchet L, Landesman SH. *Antimicrob Agents Chemother* 1984; **26**: 110–111.

(27) Simpson IN, Harper PB, O'Callaghan CH. *Antimicrob Agents Chemother* 1980; **17**: 929–936.

(28) Roy C, Segura C, Tirado M, Reig R, Hermida M, Teruel D, Foz A. *Eur J Clin Microb* 1985; **4**: 146–147.

(29) Breeze AS, Obaseiki-Ebor EE. *J Antimicrob Chemother 1983;* **12**: 459–467.

Management of urinary tract infection in children and adolescents

I. BOLLGREN

*Department of Paediatrics, Karolinska Institute,
Sachs' Children's Hospital, Stockholm, Sweden*

Introduction

The aims of management of urinary tract infection (UTI) in children and adolescents are two-fold: (a) to prevent development of renal damage and (b) to relieve acute discomfort. Renal scar formation occurs almost exclusively in small children with pyelonephritis. Children over 4 years of age are usually not at risk of renal scarring in previously undamaged kidneys. At this age, lower UTIs predominate and the main problem is the proneness to recurrent infections, which is characteristic of many girls.

Since, in many respects, upper and lower UTIs during childhood present different clinical entities, this survey will discuss them separately. However, it has to be stated that, at present, there is no perfect method to determine the localization of urinary infections. Fever is considered indicative of renal involvement. C-reactive protein (CRP) is discriminative between symptomatic upper and lower UTI, but is less reliable in asymptomatic bacteriuria (ABU) (1). In doubtful cases, assessment of maximal renal concentration capacity is warranted.

Pathogenesis of UTI

UTI is generally assumed to be ascending, with the infecting organism (mostly *Escherichia coli*) emanating from the bowel flora (2,3). Two theories have been presented to explain the preponderance of *E. coli* in UTI. The prevalence theory proposes that this is due to the mere predominance of *E. coli* in the faecal flora, which implies that there are defects in the normal host defence system which permit faecal bacteria to ascend the urinary tract. The special pathogenicity theory assumes that *E. coli* carry some special uropathogenic property. A recent advance, supporting this theory, is the finding that uropathogenic *E. coli* carry special fimbriae that adhere to uroepithelium (4).

Recent advances in the treatment of urinary tract infections, edited by F. H. Schröder, 1985: Royal Society of Medicine Services International Congress and Symposium Series No. 97, published by Royal Society of Medicine Services Limited.

In the light of present knowledge, it seems likely that an interaction between host factors and bacterial virulence factors is responsible for the establishment of bacteria in the urinary tract. The clinical expression and level of infection, however, depend on which of these two factors is predominant.

Host factors

Age and sex play a role in the infections. Small children are apt to get febrile infections and the rate of infection is highest during the first year of life. This suggests either that a sensitive population is infected early in life or that resistance gradually develops. Boys are distinguished from girls in that infections occur mainly during the first 6 months of life, the recurrence rate is low, and the spectrum of infecting bacteria is somewhat different.

In healthy girls, a local defence system is apparently acting in the periurethral and introital areas. Girls and women who are prone to recurrent infections have a periurethral colonization of enteric Gram-negative rods which precedes the ascendance of infection (5,6). This contrasts with non-susceptible females who, after 4 years of age, have no Gram-negative rods in this region (7). A more abundant flora of anaerobic Gram-negative rods is also found in the infection-prone group (8). Uroepithelial cells from infection-prone girls and women also have an increased ability to adhere to Gram-negative rods as well as other bacteria (9,10,11). Another factor is efficient bladder emptying, which is an important mechanism for clearance of bacteria, as will be discussed below.

Bacterial virulence factors

Many virulence factors for E. coli have been proposed, such as O-serotype, certain K-antigens and haemolytic activity, but definite proof of their importance has not been established. The role of bacterial adhesion in the pathogenesis of UTI is a fairly new field of research. Bacterial adhesion to a mucosal surface is the first step in the establishment of various infections (12). Even in the urinary tract, efficient adhering mechanisms are apparently operative, permitting the bacteria to resist the clearing effect of the urinary flow.

E. coli isolated from patients with pyelonephritis adhere significantly better to uroepithelium as compared with E. coli of faecal origin (13). Källenius and Möllby (14) showed that this adhesion to uroepithelium correlates with a mannose-resistant haemagglutination of human erythrocytes which is connected with the P-blood group system. (Erythrocytes from individuals of the rare p-phenotype, that lack the P-group antigens, are not agglutinated by pyelonephritogenic E. coli.) This association enabled the receptor on the erythrocyte and the uroepithelium binding the E. coli to be characterized, the active site being [α-D-Gal-(1-4)-β-D-Gal] (15). The bacterial adhesin responsible for binding to this receptor is known as P-fimbriae. P-fimbriated E. coli are found in the urine of 90% of children with acute febrile UTI. The incidence in recurrent UTI is about 20%, and about 10% in faeces from healthy children (16). In studies of experimental pyelonephritis in the monkey, it was found that P-fimbriated E. coli caused ascending pyelonephritis, while other E. coli could not (17,18). This suggests that P-fimbriation of E. coli is an important virulence factor. However, other factors also appear to be contributory, since the majority of children having a faecal colonization with P-fimbriated *E. coli* never acquire infection.

Acute pyelonephritis

Febrile UTI mainly affects small children, with a male predominance during the first 6 months of life, whereas later on girls are in the majority. Symptoms are usually diffuse in the youngest children, with fever as the most prominent symptom. Loin pain is generally not seen before 4 years of age. Diagnosis is based on a positive urine culture in combination with leucocyturia. A positive urine culture without leucocyturia should raise the suspicion of contamination of the urine specimen. In doubtful cases, it may be preferable to perform a bladder puncture. A positive CRP confirms renal involvement. In 135 cases of childhood pyelonephritis, 130 were caused by *E. coli*, 90% of which were P-fimbriated (Hammarlind *et al.*, unpublished work).

Small children with pyelonephritis are at risk of renal scarring, which subsequently may cause hypertension or chronic renal failure in adult life. The risk of scar formation is reported to be about 5% in promptly treated pyelonephritic patients (19). In the case of ABU the incidence is considerably higher, suggesting that early infections were undiscovered (20). The risk factors for permanent renal damage are low age, obstruction, gross reflux and delay in commencement of treatment. Hopefully, with an increased awareness of these risk factors, the incidence of permanent renal damage will fall.

The youngest children run the greatest risk of parenchymal damage. After 4 years of age the incidence of new scars is minimal (19). Infections complicated by obstruction to the urinary flow rapidly become deleterious if not efficiently treated. In addition to alertness for the clinical signs of obstruction (protracted fever, uncommon infecting organisms, palpable mass), ultrasonography is a reliable method in the acute phase of pyelonephritis to demonstrate dilatation of the collecting system (Table 1). In cases with dilatation, the investigation is completed by acute i.v. pyelography; further management is decided in co-operation with a urologist.

Table 1

Findings in 12 children with hydronephrosis at acute renal ultrasonography in a study comprising 140 children, consecutively scanned during the acute phase of pyelonephritis

Number of children	Acute excretion urography	Micturition cystography	Treatment and follow-up
1	Uretero-pelvic obstruction	0	Surgical correction
1	Duplication with ectopia of ureter	0	Heminephrectomy
4	Dilatation, normal excretion	Reflux grade IV–V	Conservative
5[a]	Dilatation, normal excretion	0	Conservative, successive regress of dilatation
1[a]	Dilatation, delayed excretion	0	Acute pyelostomy, restitution of kidney function, regress of dilatation

[a]Interpreted as functional hydronephrosis on basis on infection, (cf. reference 17 and Bollgren and Hammarlind, unpublished work).

Vesico-ureteral reflux (VUR) may be physiological in small children but the prevalence then rapidly decreases (21). It has been a matter of controversy whether scar formation is associated with VUR in the absence of infection. Accumulated data indicate that, in the absence of obstruction, infection is a necessary factor for new scars to develop (22). Renal scarring is mainly linked with gross reflux, i.e. dilatation of the collecting system, and especially with the presence of intrarenal reflux (IRR) (23). The pathophysiology of IRR has been thoroughly elucidated in experiments on pigs (24). New scars may also appear without demonstrable persistent reflux (25). Roberts' experiments in monkeys (17) suggest that transient pyelorenal reflux may occur during infection. He shows that some P-fimbriated E. coli strains cause ureteral paralysis, resulting in an increased ureteral pressure and pyelorenal backflow. Delay in starting treatment apparently has a great impact on scar formation. The incidence of scar formation in children with inadequately treated infections was found to be four times as high as in children receiving prompt therapy (25). Experiments in rats also show that the grade of scar formation is directly related to delay in commencing treatment (26). In conclusion, early diagnosis and prompt therapy are conceivably the most efficient way to prevent renal damage in childhood pyelonephritis. Treatment is discussed below.

The radiological investigation, including i.v. pyelography and micturition cystography, is generally performed within 1–2 months after diagnosis of uncomplicated infection. Renal ultrasonography is increasingly employed. Besides visualizing dilatation of the collecting system, this technique is also being increasingly used for primary screening of renal parenchyma, replacing urography in selected cases (27). Ultrasonography does not appear to be a reliable substitute for micturition cystography. Radionuclide techniques, however, are gradually tending to replace conventional radiology.

Follow-up includes repeated checks for recurrent bacteriuria during the next year, and a complete scan of kidney growth. Boys rarely have recurrences, but girls show a recurrence rate of about 25% during the first year after infection. Children with gross reflux and/or scars are subject to a long-term follow-up, usually in collaboration with a urologist. Recent comprehensive studies on the management of gross VUR seem to favour a conservative approach with long-term chemoprophylaxis, in preference to surgery (28).

Non-febrile, lower UTI

Non-febrile, lower UTI mainly affects children over 3–4 years of age with a female predominance. It presents with a wide range of symptoms, varying from a troublesome, acute onset to completely asymptomatic cases. In children with a single episode of cystitis, bacterial virulence factors play a role. In 57 patients with a first-time, symptomatic lower UTI, half of the E. coli strains were P-fimbriated (Lidefelt et al., unpublished work). (This contrasts with previous findings, mainly among girls with recurrent infections, of 20% of E. coli being P-fimbriated.) In older children, age-dependent host factors should, hypothetically, limit infection with P-fimbriated E. coli to the bladder.

In the large group of girls susceptible to recurrent infections, host factors appear to be decisive in the occurrence of UTI, allowing various enterobacteria to gain access to the urinary tract. The importance of periurethral colonization and the mucosal barrier has been discussed above. A careful record of the history of micturition habits is important in the management of UTI-prone girls. Many girls retain small volumes of residual urine in the bladder after voiding, which help to maintain bacteriuria (29). In a group of young girls, the bacteriuria is part of a bladder dysfunctional syndrome which presents with wetting during daytime and when squatting, and accompanied by urgency both during infection and during infection-free intervals (30). These symptoms prompt for a careful investigation, including radiology, of the urinary tract. Assessment of bladder function by measurements of intravesical pressure may further elucidate the problem. The bacteriuria usually seems to be secondary to a defective bladder emptying, analogous to UTIs in neurogenic bladders. However, experiments in cats have given evidence that bacterial endotoxins inhibit neurotransmission in the bladder, causing disturbances of the bladder contractions (31). This finding may indicate that long-standing bacteriuria may, in some cases, be deleterious to bladder function.

However, the majority of infection-prone girls show milder symptoms with successive recurrences and have no problems with bladder function. This type of infection is considered fairly innocuous, and in many cases it seems justified not to treat asymptomatic recurrences, provided that the radiological investigation is normal and renal involvement is excluded. Some girls exhibit a decreased proneness at puberty which may be partly explained by alterations of the indigenous bacterial flora of the urethral orifice due to hormonal influences; however, a returning proneness is often observed at the start of sexual activity.

Asymptomatic bacteriuria in children, disclosed by screening, has been a matter of much concern (32). This population shows a high rate of renal scarring (about 25%), evidently resulting from renal damage during early childhood. As in symptomatic infections, new scars do not develop after 4 years of age. A large proportion of infections disappear spontaneously. The present attitude is generally to leave untreated those girls who show no signs of renal involvement.

The urethral syndrome, well known in adult women, also affects girls. In girls presenting with symptoms of cystitis, including pyuria, 20% were found to have sterile urine, in a study including 97 children (Lidefelt, unpublished work). The aetiology has not been well defined but is probably multifactorial.

Treatment of UTI

In the management of UTI the emphasis is on the elimination of bacteria by the use of chemotherapeutics. In selected cases, long-term suppressive therapy with antimicrobials is warranted. In cases with obstructive malformations and, rarely, in cases of gross VUR, surgical correction may be decisive to prognosis. Girls prone to recurrent infections should be instructed on bladder emptying as a complement to the pharmacological treatment. Asymptomatic bacteriuria is often preferably left untreated. Recent research on the pathogenesis of UTI has generated new approaches to its management. Experiments in monkeys have shown that immunization with a P-fimbriae antigen has a protective effect (33). However, the clinical implication of this for childhood UTI is, for the present, uncertain. Treatment of UTI during the neonatal period deserves special considerations, details of which are given elsewhere (34).

Pharmacological treatment

General considerations

The choice of antimicrobial for the treatment of UTI includes the following aspects:
(a) Pharmacokinetic properties.
(b) Antibacterial activity against UTI pathogens, particularly important because of ecological effects on bowel bacterial flora.
(c) Adverse drug reactions (35,36,37).

Pharmacokinetics

In order to eliminate bacteria from the urinary tract, it is important that an effective antimicrobial concentration in the urine is achieved. Drugs attaining inhibitory levels in the renal parenchyma, such as amoxycillin and co-trimoxazole, are usually recommended for the treatment of pyelonephritis and are necessitated in patients with obstruction, anatomical or functional, to the urinary flow. Clinical experience shows that uncomplicated cases of pyelonephritis with intact host defence mechanisms are safely cured by chemotherapies which give high urinary levels only, such as the short-acting sulphonamides or nitrofurantoin macrocrystals.* High serum levels of antibiotic are necessary in those rare cases with bacteraemia. Antimicrobial concentrations in the bowel are important with respect to their effects on bowel bacterial ecology, as is discussed below. Nitrofurantoin macrocrystals has the unique property of being specific to the urinary tract, thus preventing faecal flora intact, and being bactericidal to common UTI pathogens (38).

Antibacterial activity

A wide range of antimicrobials is effective against *E. coli*, the most common UTI pathogen, and the bacteriuria is usually promptly eradicated. The relatively large proportion of infections caused by *Proteus* (in boys) and *Staphylococcus saprophyticum* (in adolescent girls) may influence the choice of drug.

   In recurrent infections, as well as in long-term suppressive antimicrobial therapy, most problems concern the influence of therapy on faecal flora. Agents with high concentrations in the gut tend to select for antibiotic-resistant strains or cause development of acquired resistance in previously sensitive strains. Ampicillin and, to a lesser extent, amoxycillin often select for ampicillin-resistant *Klebsiella* and sulphonamides usually cause a transient predominance of sulphonamide-resistant *E. coli* in the bowel. Development of antimicrobial resistance reflects the duration of therapy and is most pronounced in populations exposed to heavy antibiotic pressure, e.g. in urological units. Reports on the rapid development of trimethoprim resistance in geriatric wards have led to recommendations to restrict the use of this drug to

*Nitrofurantoin macrocrystals, originated by Norwich Eaton Pharmaceuticals, Inc., is distributed under the following registered trade marks: Benelux, Furadantine MC®; West Germany, Furadantin Retard®; USA, Canada and UK, Macrodantin®; France, Furadantine®; Latin America, Macrodantina®.

ambulant practice, which has aided in preserving a high sensitivity to trimethoprim. Since nitrofurantoin macrocrystals is urinary tract specific, it does not reach effective concentrations in the gastrointestinal tract and thus has the advantage of producing minimal alterations in the patient's own resident gut flora. Co-trimoxazole and trimethoprim eradicate a large proportion of rectal and periurethral *E. coli* but often leave a colonization with enterococci and staphylococci. The elimination of *E. coli* may be an advantage in prevention of UTI but reinfections with these other organisms are not rare.

Adverse reactions

Caution about toxic side-effects of drugs warrants a restrictive use of antibiotics in children, and it is certainly a wise policy to prescribe a limited number of substances. Drugs which have a selective activity against bacterial metabolism and which do not interfere with human metabolism, e.g. β-lactam antibiotics, are the most non-toxic antibiotics.

In fact, children seldom show serious adverse reactions to UTI antimicrobials, as compared with adults. Some of the reasons for this difference are that drugs are more appropriately prescribed according to body weight, that interference from concomitant use of other drugs seldom occurs, and that renal function is usually intact in children. Serious reactions against, for example, nitrofurantoin, such as pulmonary complications, are extremely rare in children. Co-trimoxazole, widely used in paediatric practice, has recently been put under careful scrutiny owing to reports on serious adverse reactions (Table 2). Even with this drug, however, adverse reactions mainly occur in elderly patients and only rarely in children and adolescents. Most adverse reactions to co-trimoxazole are attributed to the sulphonamide component, which gives grounds for an alternative use of trimethoprim alone (39).

Serious reactions to sulphonamides have led to a significant reduction in the prescription of this drug, which previously was a drug of first choice in the management of childhood UTI. Short-acting sulphonamides are probably less

Table 2

Adverse reactions to co-trimoxazole reported 1972–1984 to Swedish Adverse Drug Reactions Advisory Committee (SADRAC), National Board of Health and Welfare, 1985[a]

Reported number of cases	1234[b]
Females	68%
Median age	60–69 years
Reported number of reactions	1721
Serious reactions	20%
No. of deaths	23
Females	73%
Median age	79 years

[a]From: Swedish Board of Health and Welfare Committee on Side Effects of Pharmaceutical Preparations (The Drugs Side Effects Committee) (1985) Trimethoprim-sulphamethoxazole — a review. Report No. 44.
[b]Incidence rate of 4–6 reports per 10 000 10-day courses.

frequently associated with adverse reactions than are those with a long excretion time. Newer antibiotics, like pivmecillinam (amdinocillin pivoxil) and the cephalosporins, still make up only a minor part of the drugs used for the treatment of UTI in children and as yet have not been the subject of many reports on adverse reactions in children.

Treatment of acute pyelonephritis

Co-trimoxazole or amoxycillin can usually be recommended, provided that antibiotic sensitivity tests accord, since these substances are considered bactericidal and achieve renal parenchymal concentrations. Pivmecillinam or cephalosporins are alternative drugs of choice (Table 3). A 10-day course of treatment is the rule; longer full-dose periods have no advantage and increase the risk of side-effects. Shorter regimens may suffice, but controlled studies concerning optimal length of therapy are still lacking. Oral administration is usually preferable but parenteral administration may be necessary in vomiting children. Pyelonephritis complicated with obstruction of the urinary tract should be managed in co-operation with a urologist. In children below 1 year of age who have completed the full course of systemic therapy, we find it convenient to follow with suppressive low-dose nitrofurantoin macrocrystals or trimethoprim until micturition cystography has been performed for diagnosis of reflux. The suppressive long-term regimen in established cases of gross reflux is discussed below.

Table 3
Therapy of febrile urinary infection

	Dose/ kg/24 h	No. of doses/24 h
Trimethoprim/sulphonamide[a]	6 mg/30 mg	2
Amoxycillin[a]	40 mg	3
Cephalexin[a]	50 mg	3

[a]Duration of therapy 7–10 days.

Non-febrile lower UTI

Nitrofurantoin macrocrystals is the drug of choice, being well tolerated and exerting little influence on bowel ecology and, accordingly, with a low incidence of resistant strains. Nausea and vomiting are usually only minor problems with a dose not exceeding 3 mg/kg body w/day. Trimethoprim is an alternative choice, but treatment periods should be as short as possible in order to avoid disturbances of bowel ecology and adverse reactions to the drug. A 5-day course usually relieves symptoms and eradicates bacteriura in symptomatic lower UTI. Three days of treatment or even single-dose therapy with, for example, short-acting sulphonamide adequately eliminates bacteriuria in girls prone to recurrent infections, analogous to results in adult women (40,41). Duration of treatment does not seem to affect the recurrence rate. Whether acute first-time cystitis in children is efficiently treated with single-dose therapy remains to be shown (Table 4).

Asymptomatic bacteriuria in schoolgirls is preferably left untreated, provided that there is no renal involvement (32). Correspondingly, it sometimes seems justified to

Table 4

Therapy of afebrile symptomatic urinary infections (single and recurrent)

	Dose/ kg/24 h	No. of doses/24 h
Nitrofurantoin macrocrystals[a]	3 mg	3
Trimethoprim[a]	6 mg	2
Sulphonamide (short-acting)[a]	100 mg	3
Amoxycillin[a]	20 mg	3
Trimethoprim/sulphonamide[a]	6 mg/30 mg	2

[a]Duration of therapy 1, 3 or 5 days. Three days are probably sufficient for single infections with long intervals. For frequently recurring infections one single dose or 1-day treatment is often sufficient for elimination of infection.

omit treatment of asymptomatic recurrences in infection-prone girls with normal urological findings.

Long-term suppression

This is indicated in (a) small children with gross VUR or in recurrent episodes of pyelonephritis and in (b) girls prone to frequent recurrences of UTI. Children with gross reflux or recurrent episodes of pyelonephritis are given prophylaxis to prevent progressive renal scar formation. Nitrofurantoin macrocrystals administered in a daily dose of 1 mg/kg body wt is the drug of choice. Trimethoprim and co-trimoxazole are alternative drugs. Boys often have a preputial colonization with *Proteus mirabilis* that *a priori* may be resistant to nitrofurantoin macrocrystals, which warrants suppressive therapy with either of the latter drugs. The duration of suppressive therapy is determined by the outcome of subsequent radiology. In cases of persistent gross reflux or new scars, prophylaxis may last for years. In selected cases, surgical correction is judged to be a better alternative.

In girls with frequent symptomatic recurrences of UTI, long-term suppressive therapy is sometimes justified, not on account of the risk of scar formation, but with regard to the patient's convenience. Signs of bladder dysfunction, e.g. daytime wetting or significant residual bladder urine, strengthen the indications for suppression. Nitrofurantoin macrocrystals is the drug of choice, with trimethoprim as the best alternative. The lowest possible dose should be tested; a single dose every second night often works. The length of suppressive therapy varies according to the individual, but treatment periods of about 6 months seem advisable (Table 5). The importance of efficient bladder emptying is emphasized.

Table 5

Suppressive therapy against reinfection

	Dose/ kg/24 h	No. of doses/24 h
Nitrofurantoin macrocrystals[a]	1 mg	1
Trimethoprim[a,b]	1–2 mg	1
Trimethoprim/sulphonamide[a,c]	1–2 mg/5–10 mg	1

[a]Duration of therapy empiric.
[b]In infants with gross reflux trimethoprim is preferred.
[c]Only for prevention of renal damage.

Conclusion

The management of UTI in children and adolescents is, on the one hand, simple, in that the infection involves a relatively small number of well recognized organisms; but it is complicated by the emergence of resistance, by structural defects of the urinary tract, and by the likelihood of persistent recurrences and the risk of permanent renal damage.

The choice of agent for treating UTI in this population—as in a wide range of patients—is governed by the factors of pharmacokinetics (bactericidal concentrations of the drug in the urinary tract only); antibacterial activity (low or no emergence of resistance to therapy); and a low incidence of adverse reactions.

None of the agents available for use in the management of UTI can be described as ideal. Nevertheless, nitrofurantoin macrocrystals presents a good profile when assessed against the parameters of UTI management outlined above, and is the drug of choice in non-febrile lower UTI and in long-term suppressive therapy in small children with gross VUR or recurrent pyelonephritis and in girls prone to frequent recurrences of UTI. We also use nitrofurantoin macrocrystals as low dose suppressive therapy, following short-term treatment of acute pyelonephritis, until reflux has been assessed.

References

(1) Lindberg U, Jodal U, Hanson LÅ, Kaijser B. Asymptomatic bacteriuria in schoolgirls: IV. Difficulties of level diagnosis and the possible relation to the character of infecting bacteria. *Acta Paediatr Scand* 1975; **64**: 574–580.
(2) Turck M, Petersdorf RG. The epidemiology of non-enteric *Escherichia coli* infections: Prevalence of serological groups. *J Clin Invest* 1962; **41**: 1760–1765.
(3) Vosti KL, Goldberg LM, Monto AS, Rantz LA. Host-parasite interaction in patients with infections due to *Escherichia coli*. I. The serogrouping of *E. coli* from intestinal and extra intestinal sources. *J Clin Invest* 1964; **43**: 2377–2385.
(4) Källenius G, Möllby R. Adhesion of *Escherichia coli* to human periurethral cells correlated to mannose-resistant agglutination of human erythrocytes. *FEMS Microbial Letter* 1979; **5**: 295–299.
(5) Bollgren I, Winberg J. The periurethral aerobic bacterial flora in girls highly susceptible to urinary infections. *Acta Paediatr Scand* 1976; **65**: 81–87.
(6) Stamey TA, Timothy M, Millar M, Mihara G. Recurrent urinary infections in adult women. The role of introital enterobacteria. *Calif Med* 1971; **115**: 1–18.
(7) Bollgren I, Winberg J. The periurethral bacterial flora in healthy boys and girls. *Acta Paediatr Scand* 1976; **65**: 74–80.
(8) Bollgren I, Nord CE, Pettersson L, Winberg J. Periurethral anaerobic microflora in girls highly susceptible to urinary infections. *J Urol* 1981; **125**: 715–720.
(9) Fowler JE Jr, Stamey TA. Studies of introital colonization in women with recurrent urinary infections VII. The role of bacterial adherence. *J Urol* 1977; **117**: 472–476.
(10) Källenius G, Winberg J. Bacterial adherence to periurethral epithelial cells in girls prone to urinary tract infections. *Lancet* 1978; **2**: 540–543.
(11) Svanborg-Edén C, Jodal U. Attachment of *Escherichia coli* to urinary sediment epithelial cells from urinary tract infection-prone and healthy children. *Infect Immun* 1979; **26**: 837–840.
(12) Beachey EH (ed). *Bacterial adherence, receptors and recognition* (series B). London and New York: Chapman and Hall, 1980; vol. 6.

(13) Svanborg-Edén C, Hanson LÅ, Jodal U, Lindberg U, Sohl Akerlund A. Variable adherence to normal human urinary-tract epithelial cells of *Escherichia coli* strains associated with various forms of urinary tract infections. *Lancet* 1976; **2**: 490–492.

(14) Källenius G, Möllby R. Adhesion of *Escherichia coli* to human periurethral cells correlated to mannose-resistant agglutination of human erythrocytes. *FEMS Microbiol Letter* 1979; **5**: 295–299.

(15) Källenius G, Möllby R, Svenson SB, *et al*. The P^k antigen as receptor for the haemagglutinin of pyelonephritic *Escherichia coli*. *FEMS Microbiol Letter* 1980; **7**: 297–302.

(16) Källenius G, Möllby R, Svenson SB, *et al*. Occurrence of P-fimbriated *Escherichia coli* in urinary tract infections. *Lancet* 1981; **2**: 1369–1372.

(17) Roberts JA. Experimental pyelonephritis in the monkey. III. Pathophysiology of ureteral malfunction induced by bacteria. *Invest Urol* 1975; **13**: 117–120.

(18) Roberts JA, Kaack B, Källenius G, Möllby R, Svenson SB, Winberg J. Receptors for pyelonephritogenic Escherichia coli in primates. *J Invest Urol* 1984; **131**: 163–168.

(19) Winberg J, Bergström T, Jacobsson B. Morbidity, age and sex distribution, recurrences and renal scarring in symptomatic urinary tract infection in childhood. *Kidney Int* 1975; **8** (suppl): 101–106.

(20) McLachlan MSF, Meller ST, Verrier Jones R, *et al*. Urinary tract in schoolgirls with covert bacteriuria. *Arch Dis Child* 1975; **50**: 253–258.

(21) Köllerman MW, Ludwig H. Uber den vesico-ureteralen Reflux beim normalen Kind im Säuglings- und Kleinkindalter. *Z Kinderheilk* 1967; **100**: 185–191.

(22) Smellie JM, Normand ICS. Bacteriuria, reflux and renal scarring. *Arch Dis Child* 1975; **50**: 581–585.

(23) Rolleston GL, Maling TMJ, Hodson CJ. Intrarenal reflux and the scarred kidney. *Arch Dis Child* 1974; **49**: 531–539.

(24) Ransley PG, Risdon RA. Renal papillary morphology and intrarenal reflux in the young pig. *Urol Res* 1975; **3**: 105–109.

(25) Winberg J, Bollgren I, Källenius G, Möllby R, Svensson SB. Clinical pyelonephritis and focal renal scarring. A selected review of pathogenesis, prevention and prognosis. *Fine Pediatric Nephrology Pediatr Clins N Am* 1982; **29**: 801–814.

(26) Miller T, Phillips S. Pyelonephritis: the relationship between infection, renal scarring and antimicrobial therapy. *Kidney International* 1981; **19**: 654.

(27) Leondias JC, McCauley RGK, Klauber GC, Fretzayas AM. Sonography as a substitute for excretory urography in children with urinary tract infection. *Am J Radiol* 1985; **144**: 815–819.

(28) Birmingham Reflux Study Group. A prospective trial of operative versus non-operative treatment of severe vesico-ureteric reflux: 2 years observation in 96 children. In: Hodson CJ, Heptinstall RH, eds. *Contributions to nephrology: reflux nephropathy update*. Basle: Karger, 1984; 169–185.

(29) Lindberg U, Bjure J, Haugstvedt S, Jodal U. Asymptomatic bacteriuria in schoolgirls. III. Relation between residual urine volume and recurrence. *Acta Paediatr Scand* 1975; **64**: 437–440.

(30) van Gool JD, Kuijten RH, Donckerwolcke RA, Messer AP, Vijverberg M. Bladder-sphincter dysfunction, urinary function and vesico-ureteral reflux with special reference to cognitive bladder training. In: Hodson CJ, Heptinstall RH, eds. *Contributions to Nephrology: Reflux Nephropathy Update*. Basle: Karger, 1984; 190–210.

(31) Nergårdh A. The functional role of adrenergic receptors in the outlet region of the urinary bladder. *Scand J Urol Nephrol* 1974; **8**: 100.

(32) Verrier-Jones K, Asscher AW. Asymptomatic and covert bacteriuria. In: Francois B, Perrin P, eds. *Urinary infection. Insights and prospects*. London, Boston, Durban, Singapore, Sydney, Toronto, Wellington: Butterworths, 1983; 35–45.

(33) Svenson SB, Källenius G, Korkonen T, *et al.* Initiation of clinical pyelonephritis — the role of P-fimbriae-mediated bacterial adhesion. In: Hodson CJ, Heptinstall RH eds. *Contributions to nephrology: reflux nephropathy update* . Basle: Karger, 1984; 252–272.

(34) Klein JO. Bacterial infections of the urinary tract. In: Remington JS, Klein JO, eds. *Infectious diseases of the fetus and newborn infant*. Philadelphia and London: W. B. Saunders, 1983; 771–781.

(35) Fabre J, Dayer P, Fox HT. Antimicrobial therapy of urinary infections: extrarenal adverse reactions and side effects. In: Francois B, Perrin P, eds. *Urinary infection: insights and prospects*. London and Boston: Butterworths, 1983; 237–254.

(36) Garrod LP, Labert HP, O'Grady FO. *Antibiotic and chemotherapy* (5th edn). Edinburgh, London, Melbourne and New York: Churchill Livingstone, 1981.

(37) Speller DCE. Chemotherapy of urinary tract infection: microbiological and pharmacological aspects. In: Francois B, Perrin P, eds. *Urinary infection. Insights and prospects*. London and Boston: Butterworth, 1983; 255–270.

(38) Stamey TA, Condy M, Mihara G. Prophylactic efficacy of nitrofurantoin macrocrystals and trimethoprim-sulphamethoxazole in urinary infections. *N Engl J Med* 1977; **296**: 780–783.

(39) Brumfitt W, Hamilton-Miller JMT. Co-trimoxazole or trimethoprim alone? A viewpoint on their relative place in therapy. *Drugs* 1982; **24**: 453–458.

(40) Bailey RR (ed). *Single dose therapy of urinary tract infection*. Sydney: ADIS Health Science Press, 1983.

(41) Källenius G, Winberg J. Urinary tract infections treated with single dose of short-acting sulphonamide. *Br Med J* 1979; **1**: 1175–1176.

Management of urinary tract infection during pregnancy

P. J. WHALLEY

Jack A. Pritchard Professor of Obstetrics and Gynecology, University of Texas Southwestern Medical School, Dallas, Texas, USA

Urinary tract infection (UTI) during pregnancy can be a cause of significant maternal and foetal morbidity (1,2,3). For example, women who develop acute pyelonephritis more often deliver prematurely. Approximately 10% of patients have an associated bacteraemia, and endotoxic shock may occur in as many as 3% of patients. In its severest form, acute pyelonephritis and the resultant endotoxaemia can lead to multiple organ system failures with concomitant compromise of the uteroplacental-foetal unit. For these reasons, the key to the therapy of UTIs during pregnancy should be prevention.

Most women who develop acute symptomatic UTIs during pregnancy belong to a small group of patients who can be identified at their first prenatal visit as having asymptomatic bacteriuria (ASB) (4). ASB may be defined as the presence of actively multiplying bacteria somewhere within the urinary tract, excluding the distal urethra, at a time when the patient has no urinary tract symptoms. The reported frequency with which such bacteriuria can be detected during pregnancy ranges from 2 to 10%, depending primarily upon the socio-economic status of the women surveyed. The highest incidence occurs in women who are financially indigent, whereas the lowest rates occur in non-indigent, higher income groups. An additional important host factor is the presence of sickle cell haemoglobin. ASB is twice as common in pregnant women with the sickle cell trait as in pregnant women of the same socio-economic status who do not have sickle cell haemoglobin.

Approximately 20–30% of pregnant women with ASB detected early in pregnancy, if left untreated, will develop acute pyelonephritis or cystitis later in the pregnancy, usually in the third trimester (4). Furthermore, it has been amply demonstrated that treatment of these women with one of several antimicrobial agents will lower this attack rate to approximately 3%. Thus, ASB plays a central role in the aetiology of acute UTIs and the prevalence of acute pyelonephritis during pregnancy is directly related to the zeal with which an ASB screening programme is followed.

In populations where ASB is not treated, two-thirds of all women who develop acute pyelonephritis have detectable bacteriuria at the initial prenatal visit, whereas in centres where screening is routine and treatment is followed by culture surveillance,

Recent advances in the treatment of urinary tract infections, edited by F. H. Schröder, 1985: Royal Society of Medicine Services International Congress and Symposium Series No. 97, published by Royal Society of Medicine Services Limited.

P. J. Whalley

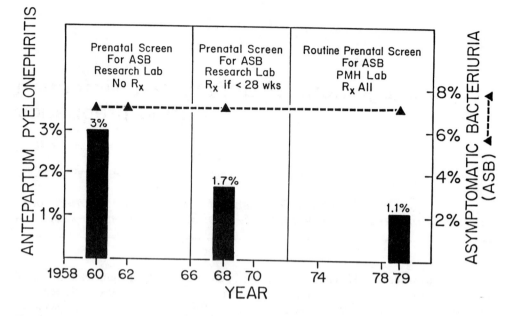

Figure 1. Decline in the incidence of antepartum pyelonephritis, 1960–1979, seen at Parkland Memorial Hospital, Dallas.

acute pyelonephritis occurs only in women who do not seek prenatal care or who develop bacteriuria after an initial sterile urine culture (less than 1% of the population). This has been our experience at Parkland Memorial Hospital, where for almost two decades all women attending our prenatal clinics have been screened for bacteriuria at their first prenatal visit followed by appropriate antimicrobial therapy and urine culture surveillance. As illustrated in Fig. 1, during this interval of time the prevalence of ASB has remained constant at 7%, whereas the incidence of acute pyelonephritis has decreased from a rate of 3% in 1960 (before screening for bacteriuria was routine) to 1·1% in 1979. A similar experience has been reported by Harris (5). On the basis of these observations we feel that the considerable maternal and foetal morbidity associated with the development of acute pyelonephritis more than justifies the effort and expense necessary to implement screening methods, particularly in populations where the incidence of ASB is high.

As noted earlier, once identified, pregnant women with proven ASB should be treated with antimicrobial agents and then monitored for recurrent bacteriuria. Because of bacterial contamination of urine during collection, the diagnosis of ASB must be based upon quantitative urine cultures. This makes it possible to distinguish between true bacterial multiplication within the urinary tract and contamination during micturition. Ordinarily, to diagnose ASB with complete assurance requires two consecutive clean-catch urine specimens each yielding the same species of micro-organism and a colony count greater than 10^5 organisms per ml of urine. However, acceptable proof of bacteriuria may vary according to clinical circumstances and during pregnancy; in the interest of time as well as expense, treatment of ASB can be started on the basis of a single urine culture. With careful patient instruction in collection technique and prompt laboratory processing, the number of false positive urine cultures can be reduced to acceptable levels. In addition, since greater than 90% of the organisms isolated are sensitive to most antimicrobial agents, organism identification and sensitivity testing are often not necessary for initial therapy. The

Table 1

Response of maternal bacteriuria to therapy with short-term and continuous antimicrobial administration

Therapy	Total no. of patients	Cured
Short-term		
First course	199	129 (65%)
Second course	70	38
Third course	32	6
		173 (87%)
Long-term		
First drug	95	83 (88%)
Second drug	12	5
		88 (93%)

expense of obtaining two urine cultures with sensitivity testing plus the consequences of delayed therapy while awaiting second culture information far outweigh the considerations of overtreatment or unnecessary treatment based on false positive results.

Because the most commonly encountered organism in ASB is *Escherichia coli*, initial selection of an antimicrobial agent is usually empirical; and a variety of agents, including sulphonamides, nitrofurantoin macrocrystals*, ampicillin, cephalosporins and, in Europe, trimethoprim, have been shown to be effective. Each of these drugs is excreted by the kidney and reaches concentrations in the urine which are greatly in excess of that required for treatment of most UTIs due to *E. coli*. However, the optimal daily dose and duration of therapy necessary to cure pregnancy bacteriuria continue to be controversial. For this reason, several years ago, we designed a study to compare the efficacy of short-*vs*-long-term continuous antimicrobial therapy for the treatment of pregnancy ASB (6). As noted in Table 1, 199 women with pregnancy bacteriuria were treated with either nitrofurantoin (Furadantine®) 200 mg/day or sulphamethizole 4 g/day in divided doses for a total of 14 days, whereas 95 women were given nitrofurantoin 100 mg/day at bedtime or sulphamethizole 4 g/day throughout gestation. Therapy for 14 days with either sulphamethizole or nitrofurantoin was effective in eradication of bacteriuria for the duration of pregnancy in 65% of patients. Following treatment with a second course of short-term therapy, this time based on sensitivity testing, another 19% of these women were cured and 3·5% responded to a third course, for a total cure rate of 87%. In the continuous therapy group, 88% of the women responded to the initial therapy becoming abacteriuric for the remainder of pregnancy. Another 5% of women responded to a second agent. Importantly, the subsequent development of acute pyelonephritis was similar in both groups—less than 3%. Thus, both treatment plans were equally effective. Because of patient convenience, low cost and a decreased potential for drug toxicity we concluded from this study that a 2-week course of therapy, when combined with continuous urine culture surveillance to detect recurrences, was preferable to continuous antimicrobial suppression throughout gestation.

Subsequently, because of the observed ease with which bacteriuria was cleared in the group of women on long-term therapy with nitrofurantoin, we treated an

*Nitrofurantoin macrocrystals, originated by Norwich Eaton Pharmaceuticals, Inc., is distributed under the following registered trade marks: Benelux, Furadantine MC®; West Germany, Furadantin Retard®; USA, Canada and UK, Macrodantin®; France, Furadantine®; Latin America, Macrodantina®.

additional 148 women with nitrofurantoin macrocrystals administered as a single 100 mg capsule at bedtime for 10 days. We chose to study this particular regimen because the vast majority of *E. coli* strains isolated from our patients with pregnancy ASB were sensitive to minimum inhibitory concentrations of nitrofurantoin ranging from 8 to 32 μg/ml, urinary concentrations easily achievable following a 100 mg oral dose of nitrofurantoin macrocrystals. In non-pregnant patients with normal renal function, 100 mg of nitrofurantoin macrocrystals result in an approximate urinary concentration of 100 μg/ml (range: 50–250 μg/ml). We reasoned that exposure of *E. coli* to such high urine concentrations for a period of 8 h while sleeping might be effective in the treatment of pregnancy ASB. The results of this study are summarized in Table 2.

Table 2

Response of maternal bacteriuria to nitrofurantoin macro-crystals[a]

Result of therapy	No. of patients
Cured for duration of gestation	93/148 (63%)
Cured, but reinfected (>6 weeks) prior to delivery	13/148 (9%)
No response or relapse (<4 weeks) prior to delivery	42/148 (28%)

[a]Macrodantin®, 100 mg h.s. for 10 days.

One course of nitrofurantoin macrocrystals was effective in eradicating bacteriuria for the remainder of pregnancy in 93 (or 63%) of the 148 women. An additional 13 women remained free of infection for at least 6 weeks, an overall bacteriologic cure rate at 6 weeks of 72%. Although serotyping of organisms was not done, the 13 recurrences were considered to be reinfections rather than relapses because of the abacteriuric time interval of 6 weeks. Eight of these women were retreated and remained abacteriuric for the duration of pregnancy. The other five were retreated and placed on suppressive therapy.

In the remaining 42 patients (28% of the total group), bacteriuria was still present following therapy or recurred within 4 weeks after therapy was completed. Cultures were not obtained during the 10-day treatment period so we were unable to determine which of these failures were due to organisms not responsive to treatment and which represented relapses with the original bacterial species. Regardless, most patients were retreated with a second and, if necessary, a third antimicrobial drug. This time the antimicrobial agent was chosen on the basis of disk sensitivity testing and given in full therapeutic doses for a total of 14 days. Twenty-four of the 42 women were subsequently cured for the duration of pregnancy. The remaining 18 patients continued to relapse. This study confirms that nitrofurantoin macrocrystals 100 mg taken at night for 10 days is an effective method for treating pregnancy bacteriuria and may be superior to other regimens because of the ease of patient compliance and lack of significant side-effects.

There is now considerable evidence that, at least in non-pregnant women, single-dose antimicrobial therapy is highly effective in the treatment of acute symptomatic UTIs which are limited to the lower urinary tract (i.e. cystitis) (7). Although the role of single-dose antimicrobial therapy in the treatment of ASB during pregnancy has not been extensively evaluated, the few studies that have been reported show an initial cure rate similar to that obtained with conventional 1–2 week therapy (8,9,10,11).

Harris and co-workers (8), using a single oral dose of 2 g of ampicillin plus 1 g, probenecid, cured 71% of 24 pregnant women with ASB. An additional 22 patients were given a single 200 mg dose of nitrofurantoin, and 20 patients were treated with 2 g of sulphisoxazole. These regimens were equally effective. Although these results appear promising, the total number of patients that have been studied is still quite small. Additional treatment trials are needed before we can determine the full impact of this form of therapy, particularly since localization studies — ureteral catheterization (12), bladder washout (13) and the fluorescent antibody test (14) — have all shown that pregnancy ASB involves the kidney in approximately 40–50% of cases. As noted earlier, at Parkland Memorial Hospital we have chosen a middle-of-the-road approach to therapy, and since 1971 all women found to have ASB at the first prenatal visit have been treated with nitrofurantoin macrocrystals, as a single 100 mg capsule at bedtime for 10 days.

The routine treatment of ASB during pregnancy and particularly daily administration of antimicrobial agents are complicated by the physician's understandable concern for the maternal and foetal side-effects of such therapy. Theoretically, any chemotherapy during pregnancy has its risks. The mother may have toxic or hypersensitivity reactions and, depending upon the amount of placental transfer, the foetus can be similarly affected. In the USA this concern is further strengthened by the fact that in *The Physicians' Desk Reference* (PDR), a compendium of prescription drugs available in the USA, there are no antimicrobial agents approved for use in pregnancy without restrictions and the package inserts of all antimicrobials carry such a warning. The obvious reasons for these 'disclaimers' is that potential drug toxicity during human embryonic and foetal development has not been adequately studied and that the teratogenic and toxic effects of a drug given during pregnancy are ultimately determined by clinical usage of the agent over time in large numbers of patients.

Nitrofurantoin has been widely used for the therapy of UTI during pregnancy since the early 1960s without reported evidence of undesirable foetal side-effects. Several years ago, Perry and co-workers (15) performed a retrospective analysis of pregnancy outcome in 101 women with ASB who received nitrofurantoin 200–400 mg daily for a mean of 49·9 days. A control group was composed of 101 women who did not have bacteriuria and did not receive drug therapy. The groups were comparable and there were no adverse effects upon Apgar scores, the occurrence of jaundice, or the incidence of congenital abnormalities. In a more recent retrospective analysis of the foetal effects of nitrofurantoin macrocrystals, Hailey and co-workers (16) reported that the incidence of foetal death, neonatal death, malformations, prematurity and low birthweight neonates born to 81 women treated with nitrofurantoin macrocrystals during 91 pregnancies was not significantly different from the general population. Jaundice was not observed in any of the infants. Similarly, our clinical experience with over 5000 pregnant women treated with 100 mg of nitrofurantoin macrocrystals daily for 10 days would suggest that such treatment is safe. These several experiences are consistent with the observed pharmacokinetics of nitrofurantoin macrocrystals.

After oral administration of the usual recommended doses of nitrofurantoin macrocrystals (200–400 mg/day), therapeutically active drug concentrations are attained only in urine and renal lymph. In individuals with normal renal function, nitrofurantoin blood levels are very low to non-existent. Although placental passage of nitrofurantoin occurs, Perry and LeBlanc (17) have reported very low to absent levels in the blood and urine of newborns and little or no nitrofurantoin was detected in amniotic fluid. It would appear from these studies that the low maternal plasma level precludes significant placental transfer so that foetal toxicity would be extremely unlikely.

Nitrofurantoin may produce a haemolytic anaemia in women whose red blood cells are markedly deficient in glucose-6-phosphate dehydrogenase (G6PD) activity. About 2% of US black women are homozygous for this enzyme deficiency and, therefore, are potential candidates for drug-induced haemolysis. However, in the past 20 years we have observed only one such case (18). An additional 10–15% of black women are heterozygous and have only a modest deficiency of G6PD. In our experience, these women are not at increased risk for the development of haemolytic anaemia when given nitrofurantoin in the usual therapeutic doses. Presumably, a drug-induced anaemia could also occur in a foetus with G6PD deficiency if the mother received nitrofurantoin as treatment for a UTI. However, this risk is more theoretical than real. As discussed above, owing to the usual low maternal plasma levels of nitrofurantoin, significant placental transfer does not occur. We have never observed a newborn with haemolytic anaemia secondary to nitrofurantoin nor have we been able to find a published report describing such a case.

In summary, since its introduction in 1953, nitrofurantoin has been widely used for the treatment of UTIs. Its reliability as an effective antimicrobial agent in the treatment of UTIs. Its reliability as an effective antimicrobial agent in the treatment of ASB in pregnancy and in the long-term suppression of bacteriuria during pregnancy is well established. The usual recommended therapeutic dose for initial therapy has been 200–400 mg/day for 7–14 days. Studies in our hospital have established that a 100 mg bedtime dose of nitrofurantoin macrocrystals given for only 10 days is equally effective. When given in this dosage there have been no adverse foetal effects, maternal side-effects have been minimal and compliance excellent.

References

(1) Gilstrap LC, Cunningham FG, Whalley PJ. Acute pyelonephritis in pregnancy: A retrospective study. *Obstet Gynecol* 1981; **57**: 409.
(2) Cunningham FG, Morris GB, Mickal A. Acute pyelonephritis of pregnancy. A clinical review. *Obstet Gynecol* 1973; **42**: 112.
(3) Cunningham FG, Leveno KJ, Hankins GDV, Whalley PJ. Respiratory insufficiency with pyelonephritis during pregnancy. *Obstet Gynecol* 1984; **63**.
(4) Whalley PJ. Bacteriuria of pregnancy. *Am J Obstet Gynecol* 1967; **97**: 723.
(5) Harris RE. The significance of eradication of bacteriuria during pregnancy. *Obstet Gynecol* 1979; **53**: 71.
(6) Whalley PJ, Cunningham FG. Short-term versus continuous antimicrobial therapy for asymptomatic bacteriuria in pregnancy. *Obstet Gynecol* 1977; **49**: 262.
(7) Bailey RR, ed. *Single dose therapy of urinary tract infections*. Sydney: ADIA Health Science Press, 1983.
(8) Harris RE, Gilstrap LC, Pretty F. Single dose antimicrobial therapy for asymptomatic bacteriuria during pregnancy. *Obstet Gynecol* 1982; **54**: 546.
(9) Bailey RR, Bishop V, Peddie RA. Comparison of single dose with a 5-day course of co-trimoxazole for asymptomatic (covert) bacteriuria of pregnancy. *Aust NZ J Obstet Gynaecol* 1983; **23**: 139.
(10) Brumfitt W, Farers M, Franklin INS. The treatment of urinary infection by means of a single dose of cephaloridine. *Postgrad Med* 1970; **46**(S): 65.
(11) Williams JD, Smith EK. Single-dose therapy with streptomycin and sulfametopyrazine for bacteriuria during pregnancy. *Br Med J* 1970; **4**: 651.
(12) Boutros P, Mourtader H, Ronald AR. Urinary infection localization. *Am J Obstet Gynecol* 1972; **112**: 379.
(13) Fairley KF, Bing AG, Adey FD. The site of infection in pregnancy bacteriuria. *Lancet* 1966; **1**: 939.

(14) Leveno KJ, Harris RE, Gilstrap LC, Whalley PJ, Cunningham FG. Bladder versus renal bacteriuria during pregnancy: Recurrence after treatment. *Am J Obstet Gynecol* 1981; **139**: 403.

(15) Perry JE, Toney JD, LeBlanc AL. Effect of nitrofurantoin on the human fetus. *Tex Rep Biol Med* 1967; **25**: 270.

(16) Hailey FJ, Fort H, Williams JC, Hammers B. Foetal safety of nitrofurantoin macrocrystals therapy during pregnancy: A retrospective analysis. *J Int Med Res* 1983; **11**: 364.

(17) Perry JE, LeBlanc AL. Transfer of nitrofurantoin across the human placenta. *Tex Rep Biol Med* 1967; **25**: 265.

(18) Pritchard JA, Scott DE, Mason RA. Severe anemia with hemolysis and megaloblastic erythropoiesis. *JAMA* 1965; **194**: 457.

The comparative safety of therapies for urinary tract infection, with special reference to nitrofurantoin

P. F. D'ARCY

Department of Pharmacy, The Queen's University of Belfast,
Northern Ireland, UK

Available agents

Anti-infective agents that are excreted primarily in the urine are useful in the treatment of uncomplicated urinary tract infections (UTIs) caused by susceptible organisms. However, because of differences in their rates of absorption and excretion, extent of protein binding, attainable urinary levels and mechanisms of action, some compounds are more effective than others. Primary systemic antibiotics include: ampicillin, tetracyclines, soluble sulphonamides, trimethoprim and co-trimoxazole (trimethoprim and sulphamethoxazole). The aminoglycosides, cephalosporins and carbenicillin are also effective but there are some restrictions to their use.

Cinoxacin, hexamine (methenamine), nalidixic acid and nitrofurantoin macrocrystals* are specific anti-infective agents which are concentrated in the urine and used only to treat UTIs. Nitrofurantoin is bactericidal against common urinary tract pathogens. Their importance lies in the management of UTIs because they are relatively non-toxic. Some are infrequently associated with the development of bacterial resistance. They may not be the drugs of first choice in upper UTIs or in the potentially septic patient with complicated UTI (1).

Relative safety

Griffin reviewed the frequency of adverse drug reactions (ADRs) reported in 12 countries in 1982 (2). The reporting of ADRs can be influenced by many factors which

*Nitrofurantoin macrocrystals, originated by Norwich Eaton Pharmaceuticals, Inc., is distributed under the following registered trade marks: Benelux, Furadantine MC®; West Germany, Furadantin Retard®; USA, Canada and UK, Macrodantin®; France, Furandantine®; Latin America, Macrodantina®.

Recent advances in the treatment of urinary tract infections, edited by F. H. Schröder, 1985: *Royal Society of Medicine Services International Congress and Symposium Series No. 97*, published by *Royal Society of Medicine Services Limited*.

may vary from one country to the next: media bias, monitoring bias, usage etc. Caution should therefore be exercised when attempting to compare data from different sources. Likewise, drug experience data from various geographical regions should not be considered homogenous. Griffin issued a warning about pooling adverse reaction data from various countries and reporting systems 62). While his warning is one of common sense, it is often ignored and data from various centres and countries are considered heterogenous and are pooled.

It is difficult, if not impossible, to assess the comparative safety of drugs used to treat UTI. Indeed, accurate knowledge of ADR rates is available for very few drugs; it is rarely developed during the clinical trial stage, and it is difficult to derive from analyses of drug-related adverse events reported to drug companies, medical journals, or even to governmental drug regulatory agencies. Indeed, few drugs have been marketed long enough to develop a reasonably accurate reaction profle for the very rare event. Such evidence as there is represents only a small and unknown fraction of the ADRs which actually occur. Furthermore, the number of patients exposed to the drug is not known, and, in the absence of accurate numerator and denominator figures, statements concerning reaction rates to individual drugs are speculative.

Although quantitative, comparative data are unobtainable, it is possible to define, at least in qualitative terms, the major adverse events that have been commonly recognized as being associated with the use of a particular drug. In an attempt to make a qualitative safety comparison between the major agents used in UTI, I have

Table 1

Urinary antimicrobial agents: comparative safety[a]

Drug	Side-effects
Ampicillins (including amoxicillin)	Diarrhoea, sensitivity reactions, angioedema anaphylactic shock, erythematous rashes in glandular fever and chronic lymphatic leukaemia, macropapular rash
Cinoxacin (azolinic acid)	Gastrointestinal, cramps, diarrhoea, hypersensitivity including rashes, peripheral and oral oedema; dizziness, headache, tinnitus, photophobia, perineal burning, changes in liver function tests.
Co-trimoxazole	Nausea, vomiting, rashes, erythema multiforma, epidermal necrolysis, eosinophilia, agranulocytosis, granulocytopenia, purpura, leukopenia, megaloblastic anaemia due to trimethoprim
Hexamine (methenamine)	Gastrointestinal frequent and painful micturition, bladder irritation, haematuria, proteinuria, rashes
Nalidixic acid	Gastrointestinal, diarrhoea, haemolysis in G6PD deficiency, allergic reactions including fever, arthralgia, eosinophilia; myalgia, muscle weakness, visual disturbances, convulsions (avoid in patients with CNS damage)
Nitrofurantoin	Gastrointestinal, rashes, peripheral neuropathy, pulmonary infiltration, haematological reactions, hepatic reactions
Tetracyclines	Nausea, vomiting, diarrhoea, super-infection with resistant organisms, tooth staining and dental hyperplasia
Trimethoprim	Nausea, vomiting, pruritus, rashes, depression of haemopoiesis

[a]Based on British National Formulary (3).

chosen to use the information in the British National Formulary as the starting point (Table 1) (3).

Anorexia, nausea and vomiting are common side-effects of urinary tract antibacterials — both systemic antibiotics and specific antibacterials. In most cases these reactions are harmless but, on occasion, may necessitate termination of treatment. Since the nature of these reactions is usually one of patient inconvenience, there are few reports of incidence and these are usually neither generalizable to other patient groups nor comparative among products.

Many urinary tract antibacterials have never become widely used or their use has declined. The reason for this is loss of efficacy through the development of resistance which may broadly be considered as an aspect of an iatrogenic disease, reduced safety, or a combination of factors (Table 2).

Table 2

Comparative safety of urinary antimicrobial drugs. The emergence of drug resistance during chronic therapy is regarded as a negative facet of safety

Nitrofurantoin	Resistance rarely develops during treatment
Cinoxacin	No information
Hexamine	Resistance does not appear to develop
Nalidixic acid	Resistance may develop rapidly
Oxolinic acid	Resistance may develop rapidly
Co-trimoxazole	Resistance developing
Trimethoprim	Resistance may develop rapidly

At one time, the soluble sulphonamides were considered to be the drugs of choice for UTI. Increasing resistance and availability of less toxic agents decreased their use. A similar decline was shown by the tetracyclines when used as urinary tract antibacterials. Hexamine (methenamine) is a urinary tract antiseptic. Its usage has declined significantly since it is only bacteriostatic and requires acidification of urine.

Cinoxacin (azolinic acid) and nalidixic acid are urinary tract agents belonging to the quinolone class. The drugs develop resistance rapidly and the class shares cross-resistance problems. Oxolinic acid, another quinolone, was marketed in the USA but was subsequently discontinued.

The ampicillins, including amoxicillin, have been used as UTI anti-infectives. They are systemic antibacterial agents with a number of indications. Resistance development to ampicillin has increased to the point where an additive, clavulanic acid, has been included in a new formulation. The systemic action of these antibacterials affects the normal gut flora and can create a bacterial as well as a fungal superinfection.

The most widely used urinary tract anti-infectives throughout the world are nitrofurantoin and co-trimoxazole. Nitrofurantoin is a urinary tract specific antimicrobial agent. Co-trimoxazole, a 5:1 combination of sulphamethoxazole and trimethoprim, is a systemic antibiotic. Trimethoprim itself is also marketed.

Co-trimoxazole

The combination of sulphamethoxazole and trimethoprim was originally developed in an attempt to reduce the adverse reactions associated with the sulphonamides and also to overcome the growing problem of resistance. Now, little more than a decade later, there is serious doubt about the adverse reaction profile of the combination, and resistance is increasingly being reported in the literature world-wide (4).

No general review or calculated incidence of major adverse reactions is available for co-trimoxazole. It is known that the combination has caused the same problems inherent to each of the components. Therefore, major reactions one might expect are various haematological toxicities, Stevens-Johnson syndrome, and pseudo-membranous colitis. Evidence based on trimethoprim alone is still too limited to allow conclusions about its relative safety. It would, however, be unwise to suspect an ADR picture markedly different from that of co-trimoxazole (5).

The Swedish Board of Health indicated an intent to review the approved indications for co-trimoxazole (6). The combination is one of the most widely used products in Sweden. The ADR Committee was considering a recommendation to remove co-trimoxazole as a first-line treatment for uncomplicated UTI. The following statement is attributed to the KabiVitrum's research director: 'These products could be removed from the market and replaced with less dangerous products' (7).

The Swedish data indicated that in 1721 ADRs co-trimoxazole was purported to be a probable or possible cause. Approximately 20% of these were considered serious: mucocutaneous syndrome, haematological and hepatic disorders, and anaphylactic reactions. 'In relation to the usage, the number of reports about serious side-effects is considerably greater for trimethoprim-sulphamethoxazole than for trimethoprim alone and other available urinary tract antibiotics. From the data available there are grounds to question, from the side-effects point of view, whether trimethoprim-sulfamethoxazole should be a preparation of first choice for uncomplicated urinary tract infections — especially in out-patient treatment' (6).

In a Danish report on blood ADRs, sulphonamide preparations and trimethoprim are considered as one class. Both trimethoprim and sulphamethoxazole are indicated as being frequently associated with aplastic anaemia, thrombocytopenia, and granulocytopenia/agranulocytosis. Sulphonamide preparations and trimethoprim are listed third in frequency for aplastic anaemia (after musculo-skeletals and cytostatics); second for thrombocytopenia after musculo-skeletals; second for granulocytopenia after musculo-skeletals; and second for agranulocytosis after musculo-skeletals (8).

The UK has also been aware of haematological problems with co-trimoxazole. It is now one of the most commonly reported causes of drug-induced thrombocytopenia. The mechanism for these reactions is still uncertain (9).

Nitrofurantoin

Of the therapies in current use, nitrofurantoin must be at the forefront of discussion simply because for over 30 years it has continued to be widely prescribed as an effective agent in the treatment of UTIs. During this time, it has withstood the rigours of constant clinical evaluation and it has successfully competed with the advent of more recent antibacterial agents. Some serious and potentially hazardous reactions to therapy have been documented and an attempt has been made in this present review, which deals largely with nitrofurantoin, to put the pulmonary, hepatic, neurological and haematological reactions associated with nitrofurantoin into perspective (10).

In the 30 years of its clinical use, nitrofurantoin has attracted a large spectrum of publications, the number of which increases constantly from year to year (Fig. 1). Some of these publications refer to adverse reactions, although most refer to positive therapeutic benefit. A number of reactions are trivial and do not present a hazard, but chronic pulmonary or hepatic effects may be life threatening and neurotoxicity,

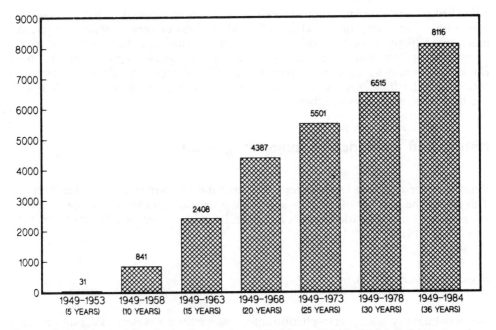

Figure 1. *Total number of nitrofurantoin publications, 1949–1984 (information from Norwich Eaton data base).*

particularly peripheral polyneuropathy, can be a serious sequel to treatment. Nitrofurantoin allegedly enters into interactions with a number of other drugs; reports of some of these have been misrepresented in the literature and have been erroneously re-cited in subsequent reviews. There is still a need for a balance sheet to be presented in which the perspective of proven clinical value and reported adverse effects of treatment are weighed against each other—a perspective of benefit versus risk.

It is extremely difficult to compare adverse reaction profiles between drugs on a quantitative basis. It is equally difficult, given the nature of prescription drug use, to build a rational profile on a single drug. The numerator must be based on reported events. Obviously, many events go unreported for a variety of reasons. The denominator must be based on known sales or courses of therapy. When a drug is available from multiple suppliers, or the duration of therapy varies widely, the denominator is limited.

In 1984, I was invited to act as an independent assessor and reviewer of the Norwich Eaton adverse reaction data base on nitrofurantoin. The purpose of the review was to ascertain a 'calculated' incidence of major adverse events. The data base contains information on all brands of nitrofurantoin (all manufacturers) and on adverse reaction reports retrieved from available published literature, from drug regulatory authorities, from case reports of studies sponsored by that company, and from information submitted to the company from any source world-wide. This became the basis for the development of the numerator. The denominator was 121 430 000 courses of therapy. This number is based on Norwich Eaton branded nitrofurantoin products in the USA since 1953 and presented as an average course of therapy. These data have now been updated to include all courses of therapy (128 000 000) and adverse reactions reported up to June 1985.

While it may be argued that the calculated incidence is inappropriate, there is nothing better or more complete. Common adverse reactions to therapy may not be published or reported once they are well known and recognized by the professional community (e.g. gastrointestinal side-effects). Serious or rare events, however, are much more likely to be published or reported to drug regulatory bodies or to the manufacturer. Therefore, the current approach via the Norwich Eaton data base (11,12) on world-wide reaction reports provides the best available information concerning the incidence of major reactions. It also provides evidence that such reactions are relatively infrequent.

Nature and incidence of major drug reactions

Reports of serious drug experiences with nitrofurantoin are summarized in Table 3. This shows the number of patients in seven major reaction categories; reaction data are presented in terms of numbers and calculated incidence world-wide from 1953 to 1985 (13,14,15).

Pulmonary reactions

Acute pulmonary reactions to nitrofurantoin may mimic a variety of conditions such as asthma (16), tracheobronchitis (17), cardiac pulmonary oedema (18), pulmonary embolism (19) and pneumonitis (20). Initial reactions usually occur within 5–10 days after starting treatment, although on subsequent treatments they may occur within a few hours. The symptoms usually subside within 24–48 h, and the chest X-ray returns to baseline within a few days.

A more chronic and insidious pulmonary infiltration associated with nitrofurantoin was first described by Sollaccio and co-workers (21) and, since that report, more than 50 other sub-acute or chronic cases have been reported, five of which were fatal (22,23,24,25,26). There was an average of 30 months of nitrofurantoin treatment before symptoms appeared (27).

The incidence of acute pulmonary reactions is 0·0009%; this has been calculated using the 1166 cases reported world-wide as the numerator and 128 000 000 courses of therapy as the denominator. Using the same system of calculation, the incidences for sub-acute and chronic pulmonary reactions are 0·00002% and 0·0002%, respectively. Miscellaneous pulmonary reactions (exact nature of reaction not defined) have an incidence of 0·0002%. Added together, these calculations indicate an overall pulmonary reaction rate of 0·001% of courses of therapy.

Hepatic reactions

Nitrofurantoin has been associated with an acute hepatocellular and cholestatic injury (28,29) but only rarely with a lesion resembling chronic active hepatitis. The first report of nitrofurantoin-induced jaundice appeared in 1961 (30); after that a few other cases of acute and, less commonly, chronic liver damage have been associated with nitrofurantoin treatment (31,32,33,34). However, little was reported on the long-term outcome of nitrofurantoin-induced liver damage until Iwarson and co-workers (35) described five patients, all women, who developed chronic liver disease after 1–3 years of continued treatment with nitrofurantoin. Liver histology was consistent with chronic

Table 3
Major adverse reactions to nitrofurantoin[a]

Reaction category	Number of patients/country					Total world-wide	Calculated incidence (%)[b]
	USA	Sweden	UK	Netherlands	Other		
Acute pulmonary reactions	342	431	110	15	268	1166	0·0009
Sub-acute pulmonary reactions	9	—	—	—	13	22	0·00002
Chronic pulmonary reactions	154	70	14	4	59	301	0·0002
Miscellaneous pulmonary reactions	7	270	—	—	7	284	0·0002
Hepatic reactions	217	20	27	18	41	323	0·0003
Neurological reactions	391	73	106	9	277	856	0·0007
Haematological reactions	394	23	13	7	71	508	0·0004

[a]Reactions filed in Norwich Eaton's data base which comprises information from literature, clinical studies, regulatory bodies and spontaneous reports from practitioners from 1953 to June, 1985.
[b]Incidence calculated using world-wide reaction figures as the numerator and 128 000 000 courses of treatment (see text) as the denominator.

active hepatitis in four of these patients, while post-necrotic cirrhosis was seen in the other case. Follow-up examinations 2–3 years after withdrawal of the drug showed marked clinical improvement and, in most cases, historical improvement also.

Sharp and co-workers reported five cases (all middle-aged to elderly women) of chronic active hepatitis, two of which were fatal (36). These cases were discussed in relation to 15 other cases reported in the literature; all of the 20 patients were women and they had taken nitrofurantoin for periods of 4 weeks to 11 years. Eighteen patients improved clinically and biochemically when the drug was withdrawn; cirrhosis occurred in four patients. Both the patients who died had taken the drug for more than 1 year and had a clinical course of progressive hepatic failure. They had continued taking nitrofurantoin despite the presence of jaundice and biochemical evidence of liver damage. Severe hepatic necrosis was found at autopsy in both patients.

The calculated incidence of hepatic reactions to nitrofurantoin is $0 \cdot 0003\%$ of treatment courses.

Neurological reactions

Nitrofurantoin has been associated with the occasional development of polyneuropathy. In an attempt to learn more about this reaction, Toole and Parrish (37) reviewed the world-wide literature. Although they were unable to ascertain the incidence of neuropathic complications among the thousands of patients who had received nitrofurantoin, they found that 137 cases of peripheral neuropathy were described in 58 reports.

In these case reports, 105 had information concerning (a) the mode and route of nitrofurantoin treatment (111 cases); (b) the length of treatment (88 cases); (c) the time relationship between the beginning of nitrofurantoin treatment and the onset of neurological symptoms (118 cases); (d) the nature of the symptoms reported (101 cases); (e) the prognosis for the neuropathy after treatment was discontinued (45 cases); and (f) the results of lumbar punctures (45 cases). However, most reports gave only sketchy information regarding blood studies, renal function or the presence of systemic abnormalities.

In the cases reviewed, nitrofurantoin was associated with a sensorimotor peripheral neuropathy, first as paresthesia and dysesthesia beginning in the distal extremities and ascending bilaterally in a 'stocking-glove' distribution. Prognosis depended on the severity of the symptoms; progression of symptoms did not seem to be related either to total dosage or to continuance of the drug after symptoms first appeared (38,39). Recovery may occur in the presence of continued renal insufficiency, chronic alcoholism with malnutrition, and anaemia (40).

The incidence of neurological reactions has been calculated to be $0 \cdot 0007\%$ of courses of therapy.

Haematological reactions

Nitrofurantoin is one of the numerous drugs which can cause, although relatively rarely, acute haemolytic anaemia in patients with intra-erythrocytic disorders, for example G6PD deficiency (41), enolase and glutathione peroxidase deficiencies (42,43). Haemolysis has also been reported in a patient who had no known enzymatic defect (44).

The calculated incidence rate of haematological reactions is $0 \cdot 0004\%$ of courses of therapy. This calculation is interesting in view of the 1971 survey of Koch-Weser and co-workers (13), which listed 13 haematological reactions to nitrofurantoin among 70 adverse reactions to 757 courses of treatment. Ten of these were eosinophilia and there was one each of haemolytic anaemia, megaloblastic anaemia and leukopenia. A later survey in Sweden (14) gave 20 cases of blood dyscrasias. Four of these were fatal (three of agranulocytosis and one of cytopenia) but in each case it was considered that a second drug (sulphamerazine with sulphaproxyline, chlorpropamide, methotrimeprazine (levopromazine), or hydrochlorothiazide) was co-responsible for the reaction. These 20 cases were not further differentiated into types of blood dyscrasias and they occurred among 921 reports of all types of reaction to nitrofurantoin.

Safety in reproductive systems

Nitrofurans, including nitrofurantoin, have been shown to produce temporary spermatogenic arrest at the stage of the primary spermatocyte in the rat testes (45,46). In studies on 36 young volunteers who took nitrofurantoin (10 mg/kg orally) for 14 days, 23 showed no significant change in sperm count or testicular biopsies and in 13 others there was a temporary decrease in sperm count but no changes could be detected in the testicular biopsies of six of these (47). Testicular biopsies in two other small studies on patients treated with nitrofurantoin were normal (48,49) and one other study showed no variation in sperm counts in such patients (50).

Later studies showed that the *in vitro* incubation of nitrofurantoin sodium with human spermatocytes led to immobilization, although the concentration of the drug (20 mg/ml) was high (51). However, none of this evidence counteracts the assurance of safety in this respect given earlier by Nelson and Bunge (47), nor indeed have there been any recent reports in the literature to question this assurance. There is little reason to fear that use of nitrofurantoin in the treatment of urinary tract infections would cause significant infertility.

Treatment of bacteriuria during pregnancy is necessary: otherwise, pyelonephritis may present a hazard for both mother and foetus (52). There is, however, a danger that any antibacterial agent may cause foetal toxicity and abnormality. In this respect, although nitrofurantoin has been shown to cross the placental barrier, it does so to a very small extent and, since maternal blood levels are so low, foetal toxicity is unlikely to occur (53). Although there is a theoretical risk of nitrofurantoin-induced haemolytic anaemia in the newborn of mothers who have G6PD deficiency (54), healthy infants have been born to such mothers (55,56), even though some of the babies had a similar deficiency (57).

Teratogenicity studies of nitrofurantoin macrocrystals in rats and rabbits have proved negative, and general reproduction and perinatal studies in rats showed no effect on fertility nor any signs of gross external or internal anomalies (58). Clinical surveys by Nelson and Forfar (59) did not detect any association between a group of antibiotics and antibacterials, including nitrofurantoin, and congenital abnormalities of the foetus.

Heinonen and co-workers (60) have contributed interesting tables of malformation risk data to Kaufman's book *Birth Defects and Drugs in Pregnancy*. They reported on 590 infants whose mothers used nitrofurantoin at any time during pregnancy. Of the 590, 83 mothers received nitrofurantoin during the first trimester. The standardized relative risk (SRR) during the first trimester (compared with 50 282 mother-child pairs) was $1 \cdot 01$. The SRR for all 590 infants was $1 \cdot 30$ with a 95% confidence interval of $0 \cdot 72 - 2 \cdot 17$. If the value of the SRR were appreciably different from unity, this would indicate an association between the drug and outcome.

All this evidence would suggest, therefore, that the risk to benefit ratio is very much on the side of the use of nitrofurantoin when it is needed to treat bacteriuria during pregnancy.

Sweden has established a classification system for drugs during pregnancy and breastfeeding. Category C is defined as 'Drugs which, in men, due to their pharmacological effects, have caused, or, for good reason can be expected to cause, a risk for the foetus and/or the newborn child without being directly teratogenic' (61). Co-trimoxazole is a Category C in Sweden. Trimethoprim as a single agent is classified as a B:3 which indicates increased foetal damage in animals, but human significance is unclear. Nitrofurantoin has been given Category A status in Sweden. This category denotes the safest drugs. Such a classification scheme has yet to be fully implemented in the USA.

The UK, the Netherlands and other countries also provide specific product labelling for drug use during pregnancy. In the UK, co-trimoxazole is contra-indicated during pregnancy. Nitrofurantoin is considered to be safe during pregnancy in both the UK and the Netherlands.

Drug interactions

Interactions between drugs are always of concern and affect the safety profile of any product. The ideal drug is one which has no significant interactions, or the interactions are so well known that management is simplified. However, if such interactions impact on patient compliance (such as the avoidance of food or drink), special attention must be given to ensure compliance.

Harmful interactions

In general, there are relatively few clinically significant drug interactions with any of the antibacterials used in UTI therapy. The most significant of these interactions occurs with co-trimoxazole.

Potentiation of warfarin sodium's anticoagulant action with concomitant use of co-trimoxazole has been reported. This interaction requires reduction of warfarin prior to treatment and a dosage readjustment when co-trimoxazole treatment is completed. There is no evidence to indicate which component of the combination is responsible for this interaction (62,63).

Co-trimoxazole has also been reported to potentiate the effects of phenytoin and increase the risk of intoxication. Both sulphamethoxazole and trimethoprim have been implicated in this reaction. It is necessary to monitor for signs of phenytoin intoxication and anticipate reduction of phenytoin if this combination is used. Inhibition of hepatic metabolism of phenytoin appears to be the mechanism involved (64).

It is important that clinicians using immunosuppressive agents such as azathioprine, mercaptopurine and methotrexate be alert to interactions with the co-trimoxazole combination. Bone marrow depression has accompanied the use of azathioprine. An *in vitro* culture indicated a potentiation of the suppressive effects of mercaptopurine (65) and there is some evidence of pancytopenia with myoblastosis as a consequence of methotrexate combination (66).

With regard to nitrofurantoin, there are relatively few documented, clinically significant drug interactions. In one case, there has been an error in the literature implicating an interaction between nitrofurantoin and alcohol. The error was based on recitation of sources without verification of the data (67). This problem is still occurring (68) and remains troublesome. In a recent review of the Norwich Eaton data base, no documented cases of a cause–effect relationship between alcohol and nitrofurantoin were found. What clinical evidence exists is anecdotal or unconfirmed by rechallenge. Nitrofurantoin suspension was marketed with 10% alcohol from its introduction in 1953 until 1966. This information, along with the results of a volunteer study to investigate the possibility of such a reaction (69), should resolve the issue.

General interactions with antacids and oral contraceptives have also been reviewed. The alleged interaction with commonly marketed antacids does not exist. The adsorption of nitrofurantoin on to magnesium trisilicate may occur, but is of doubtful clinical significance. The evidence of an interaction with oral contraceptives is little more than supposition. Evidence in the clinical literature is non-existent (10).

There is an interaction between nalidixic acid and nitrofurantoin based on *in vitro* data; the clinical significance of the study is doubtful. The clinical combination of the two products is irrational, thus making the interaction a moot issue (10).

There is a single case report of an interaction between nitrofurantoin and phenytoin. There was indirect evidence of enzyme induction and increased metabolism of phenytoin. This is different from the inhibition of hepatic metabolism of phenytoin, which is presumed to be the principal mechanism of interaction with both sulphamethoxazole and trimethoprim (10).

Beneficial interactions

Food and propantheline increase the bioavailability of nitrofurantoin. The mechanism involved is the slowing of gastric emptying. This results in slowing absorption of the drug and increasing the duration of urinary concentrations. Food has an additional 'interactive' benefit since it reduces nausea, which is the most common side-effect of nitrofurantoin and other urinary tract antibacterials.

In vitro studies by Sevag and De Courcy showed that the combined use of mepacrine (an antimutagen) with an appropriate antimicrobial drug prevented the emergence of drug-resistant strains (70,71). The mechanism involved was suggested to be a combination between mepacrine and bacterial deoxyribonucleic acid which impeded the genetic potential for the development of resistance. This concept was tested in a preliminary clinical trial by Sharda and co-workers (72) who studied the effect on UTIs of mepacrine and nitrofurantoin combined in a group of therapeutic failures. The combination eradicated a continuous *Escherichia coli/Klebsiella aerobacter* urinary infection in one case which had lasted for 120 months and this combination kept the urine sterile for 12 months. In two other cases, with frequent recurrent urinary infections, the combination sterilized the urine for 10 and 12 months, respectively. In one other case, the combination failed to affect the course of the infection.

Horwitz and co-workers confirmed both *in vitro* and *in vivo* (39 patients) that quinacrine as an adjunct to antimicrobial drug therapy (including nitrofurantoin) was more effective than the same antimicrobial agent given alone to treat UTIs (73). Later studies by Eshleman and co-workers in 149 patients with UTIs confirmed that mepacrine/antimicrobial drug (including nitrofurantoin) combinations afforded a significant therapeutic advantage over the use of antimicrobial agents alone in preventing the emergence of drug-resistant organisms (74).

Conclusions

In a recent press release, the WHO commented about drugs in pregnancy and at delivery. One paragraph is of particular interest to this symposium: '. . . animal evidence is unreliable, and evidence needs to be gathered systematically from human experience, which can only be done by keeping long-term records — for not less than 30 years — of all drugs used (including self-medication) in pregnancy' (75).

Nitrofurantoin is the oldest urinary tract antibacterial in current clinical use; it has been used for more than 30 years in the treatment of UTIs. The calculated incidence of major adverse reactions to nitrofurantoin therapy is small. Some of the adverse reactions to its use can be serious, but much is known about them and this can be regarded as a facet of safety.

Its interactions with other drugs are trivial and, as reported, they present little clinical hazard. Some of the reported interactions are anecdotal and others have been assumed on inadequate evidence.

Nitrofurantoin has a safety record for use in acute, uncomplicated UTI. No other current product has such a well documented safety profile which allows for the claim of being an ideal agent.

Acknowledgements

I thank Harvey A. K. Whitney Jr, Editor of *Drug Intelligence and Clinical Pharmacy*, for permission to cite text and information from my paper previously published in that journal.

References

(1) American Medical Association. Urinary tract antiseptics. In: *AMA drug evaluations* (5th edn). Chicago, Illinois, USA: American Medical Association, 1983; 1743–1752.

(2) Griffin JP. Survey of spontaneous adverse drug reaction reporting schemes in sixteen countries. In: *Professor James Crooks Memorial Symposium*. Dundee, Scotland, September 12, 1984; *Scrip* No. 935: 20–21.

(3) *British national formulary* No. 9. British Medical Association and The Pharmaceutical Society of Great Britain. 1985.

(4) Murray BE, Rensimer ER, DuPont HL. Emergence of high-level trimethoprim resistance in fecal *Escherichia coli* during oral administration of trimethoprim or trimethoprim-sulfamethoxazole. *N Engl J Med* 1982; **306**: 130–135.

(5) CSM (Committee on Safety in Medicines). Deaths associated with co-trimoxazole, ampicillin, and trimethoprim. *Current Problems* 1985; **15**: July.

(6) Swedish Board of Health. Trimethoprim-sulphamethoxazole — a review. Report No. 44, January, 1985.

(7) *Scrip*. Trim/sulf restrictions in Sweden. No. 966, January 21, 1985; 4.

(8) *Scrip*. Blood ADRs in Denmark. No. 1027, August 21, 1985; 20.

(9) D'Arcy PF, Griffin JP. In: *Drug-induced emergencies*, Chicago, USA: Wright & Sons Ltd, 1980; 235–236.

(10) D'Arcy PF. Nitrofurantoin. *Drug Intell Clin Pharm* 1985; **19**: 540–547.

(11) Rowles B, Worthen DB, Burns JM. Anatomy of a worldwide drug experience/publication program. In: *Worldwide drug development and scientific data management: the impact of emerging technologies and regulations.* Proceedings of the Drug Information Association, 20th Annual Meeting, San Diego: Drug Information Association, June 17–21, 1984.

(12) Worthen DB, Burns JM, Rowles B. Programme integration to support drug information and dissemination. *J Clin Hosp Pharm* (in press).

(13) Koch-Weser J, Sidel VW, Dexter M, Parish C, Finer DC, Kanarek P. Adverse reactions to sulfisoxazole, sulfamethoxazole, and nitrofurantoin. Manifestations and specific reaction rates during 2118 courses of therapy. *Arch Intern Med* 1971; **128**: 399–404.

(14) Holmberg L, Boman G, Böttiger LE, Eriksson B, Spross R, Wessling A. Adverse reactions to nitrofurantoin. Analysis of 921 reports. *Am J Med* 1980; **69**: 733–738.

(15) Penn RG, Griffin JP. Adverse reactions to nitrofurantoin in the United Kingdom, Sweden, and Holland. *Br Med J* 1982; **284**: 1440–1442.

(16) Walton CHA. Case report: asthma associated with the use of nitrofurantoin. *Can Med Assoc J* 1966; **94**: 40–41.

(17) Bayer WL, Dawson RE Jr, Kotin E. Allergic tracheobronchitis due to nitrofurantoin sensitivity. *Dis Chest* 1965; **48**: 429–430.

(18) Murray MJ, Kronenberg R. Pulmonary reactions simulating cardiac pulmonary edema caused by nitrofurantoin. *N Engl J Med* 1965; **273**: 1185–1187.

(19) Israel HL, Diamond P. Recurrent pulmonary infiltration and pleural effusion due to nitrofurantoin sensitivity. *N Eng J Med* 1962; **266**: 1024–1026.

(20) Strauss WG, Griffin LM. Nitrofurantoin pneumonia. *JAMA* 1967; **199**: 765–766.

(21) Sollaccio PA, Ribaudo CA, Grace WJ. Subacute pulmonary infiltration due to nitrofurantoin. *Ann Intern Med* 1966; **65**: 1284–1286.

(22) Ruikka I, Vaissalo T, Saarimaa H. Progressive pulmonary fibrosis during nitrofurantoin therapy. *Scand J Respir Dis* 1971; **52**: 162–166.

(23) Strandberg I, Wengle B, Fagrell B. Chronic interstitial pneumonitis with fibrosis during long-term treatment with nitrofurantoin. *Acta Med Scand* 1974; **196**: 483–487.

(24) Kursh ED, Mostyn EM, Perksy L. Nitrofurantoin pulmonary complications. *J Urol* 1975; **113**: 392–395.

(25) Sovijaervi ARA, Lemola M, Stenius B, Idaenpaeaen-Heikkilae J. Nitrofurantoin-induced acute, subacute and chronic pulmonary reactions. A report of 66 cases. *Scand J Respir Dis* 1977; **58**: 41–50.

(26) Hawley HB, Payne CB Jr, Kane KK. Nitrofurantoin pneumonitis. *Med Times* 1982; **110**: 34–39.

(27) Simonian SJ, Kroeker EJ, Boyd DP. Chronic interstitial pneumonitis with fibrosis after long-term therapy with nitrofurantoin. *Ann Thorac Surg* 1977; **24**: 284–288.

(28) Goldstein LI, Ishak KG, Burns W. Hepatic injury associated with nitrofurantoin therapy. *Am J Dig Dis* 1974; **19**: 987–998.

(29) Engel JJ, Vogt TR, Wilson DE. Cholestatic hepatitis after administration of furan derivatives. *Arch Intern Med* 1975; **135**: 733–735.

(30) Ernaelsteen D, Williams R. Jaundice due to nitrofurantoin. *Gastroenterology* 1961; **41**: 590–593.

(31) Jokela S. Liver disease due to nitrofurantoin. *Gastroenterology* 1967; **53**: 306–311.

(32) Bhagwat AG, Warren RE. Hepatic reactions to nitrofurantoin (letter). *Lancet* 1969; **ii**: 1369.

(33) Murphy KJ, Innis MD. Hepatic disorder and severe bleeding diathesis following nitrofurantoin ingestion. *JAMA* 1968; **204**: 396–397.

(34) Fagrell B, Strandberg I, Wengle B. Nitrofurantoin-induced disorder simulating chronic active hepatitis. A case report. *Acta Med Scand* 1976; **199**: 237–239.

(35) Iwarson S, Lindberg J, Lundin P. Nitrofurantoin-induced chronic liver disease: clinical course and outcome of five cases. *Scand J Gastroenterol* 1979; **14**: 497–502.

(36) Sharp JR, Ishak KG, Zimmerman HJ. Chronic active hepatitis and severe hepatic necrosis associated with nitrofurantoin. *Ann Intern Med* 1980; **92**: 14–19.

(37) Toole JF, Parrish ML. Nitrofurantoin polyneuropathy. *Neurology* 1973; **23**: 554–559.

(38) Meyer-Rienecker H, Olischer RM. Zur Nitrofurantoin-Polyneuropathie. *Nervenarzt* 1966; **37**: 410–412.

(39) Hakamies L. Die Nitrofurantoin-Polyneuropathie. *Schweiz Med Wochenschr* 1970; **100**: 2212–2218.

(40) Rubenstein CJ. Peripheral polyneuropathy caused by nitrofurantoin. In: Meyler L, Peck HM, eds. *Drug-induced diseases*. Amsterdam: Excerpta Medica Foundation, 1968; 161–164.

(41) Williams JRB. Blood dyscrasias. In: D'Arcy PF, Griffin JP, eds. *Iatrogenic diseases* (2nd edn). Oxford: University Press, 1979; 92–155.

(42) Steinberg M, Brauer MJ, Necheles TF. Acute hemolytic anemia associated with erythrocyte glutathione-peroxidase deficiency. *Arch Intern Med* 1970; **125**: 302–303.

(43) Stefanini M. Chronic hemolytic anemia associated with erythrocyte enolase deficiency exacerbated by ingestion of nitrofurantoin. *Am J Clin Pathol* 1972; **58**: 408–414.

(44) Carpel EF. Hemolysis induced by nitrofurantoin. *Pa Med* 1970; **73**: 49–50.

(45) Nelson WO, Steinberger E. The effect of furadroxyl upon the testis of the rat (abstract). *Anat Rec* 1952; **112**: 367–368.

(46) Nelson WO. Some problems of testicular function. *J Urol* 1953; **69**: 325–338.

(47) Nelson WO, Bunge RG. The effect of therapeutic dosages of nitrofurantoin (Furadantin) upon spermatogenesis in man. *J Urol* 1957; **77**: 275–281.

(48) Holloway WJ. Nitrofurantoin in urinary tract infections part 1. Nitrofurantoin revisited. *Delaware Med J* 1972; **44**: 99–104.

(49) Carroll G, Brennan RV. Furadantin. *J Urol* 1954; **71**: 650–654.

(50) Schmidt KH. Furadantin bei Harnwegsinfektionen. *Muench Med Wochenschr* 1954; **96**: 1516–1518.

(51) Albert PS, Salerno RG, Kapoor SN. Davies JE. The nitrofurans as sperm immobilizing agents. *J Urol* 1975; **113**: 69–70.

(52) Hailey FJ, Fort H, Williams JC, Hammers B. Foetal safety of nitrofurantoin macrocrystals therapy during pregnancy: a retrospective analysis. *J Int Med Res* 1983; **11**: 364–369.

(53) Perry JE, Le Blanc AL. Transfer of nitrofurantoin across the human placenta. *Tex Rep Biol Med* 1967; **25**: 265–269.

(54) Pepperell RJ. Drugs in pregnancy. *Med Int* 1983; **1**: 1636–1638.

(55) Jeannet M, Perrier CV, Toenz O. Anémie hémolytique aigue par la nitrofurantoin chez une Iranienne présentant un déficit en glucose-6-phosphate-dehydrogenase erythrocytaire. Démonstration de l'hétérozygotie de la malade par une méthode originale. *Schweiz Med Wochenschr* 1964; **94**: 939–943.

(56) Hibbard L, Thrupp L, Summeril S, Smale M, Adams R. Treatment of pyelonephritis in pregnancy. *Am J Obstet Gynecol* 1967; **98**: 609–615.

(57) Pritchard JA, Scott DE, Mason RA. Severe anaemia with hemolysis and megaloblastic erythopoiesis: a reaction to nitrofurantoin administered during pregnancy. *JAMA* 1965; **194**: 457–459.

(58) Prytherch JP, Sutton ML, Denine EP. General reproduction, perinatal-postnatal, and teratology studies of nitrofurantoin macrocrystals in rats and rabbits. *J Toxicol Environ Health* 1984; **306**: 811–823.

(59) Nelson MM, Forfar JO. Association between drugs administered during pregnancy and congenital abnormalities of the fetus. *Br Med J* 1971; **1**: 523–527.

(60) Heinonen OP, Slona D, Shapiro S. In: Kaufman DW, ed. *Birth defects and drugs in pregnancy*. Littleton, Mass., USA: Publishing Sciences Group Inc., 1977; 296–313, 422–425.

(61) Berglund F, Flodh H, Lundborg P, Sannerstedt R. In: *FASS 1985*. Uppsala, Sweden: Almqvist & Wiksell, 1985; 929–932.

(62) O'Reilly RA. Stereoselective interaction of trimethoprim-sulfamethoxazole with the separated enantiomorphs of racemic warfarin in man. *N Eng J Med* 1980; **302**: 33–36.

(63) Hassall C, Feetman CL, Leach RH, Meynell MJ. Potentiation of warfarin by co-trimoxazole. *Lancet* 1975; **2**: 1155–1156.

(64) Hansen JM, Siersbaek-Nielsen K, Skovsted L, Kampmann JP, Lumholtz B. Potentiation of warfarin by co-trimoxazole. *Br Med J* 1975; **2**: 684.

(65) Bradley PP, Warden GD, Maxwell JG, Rothstein G. Neutropenia and thrombocytopenia in renal allograft recipients treated with trimethoprim-sulfamethoxazole. *Ann Intern Med* 1980; **93**: 560–562.

(66) Kobrinsky NL, Ramsay KC. Acute megaloblastic anemia induced by high-dose trimethoprim-sulfamethoxazole. *Ann Intern Med* 1981; **94**: 780–781.

(67) Rowles B, Worthen DB. Clinical drug information: A case of misinformation (letter). *N Engl J Med* 1982; **306**: 113–114.

(68) Philp JR. Drug adverse reactions and interactions involving sulfonamides, trimethoprim, nitrofurantoin, nalidixic acid, fusidic acid, polymyxins and bacitracin. In: Petrie JC, ed. *Gastrointestinal, haematological and infectious disease therapy (clinically important adverse drug interactions)*. Amsterdam: Elsevier Science Publishers, B.V. 1985; 169–172, 184–195.

(69) Miura K, Reckendorf HK. The nitrofurans. In: Ellis GP, West GB, eds. *Progress in medicinal chemistry* (5th edn). New York: Plenum Press, 1967; 320–381.

(70) Sevag MG. Prevention of the emergence of antibiotic-resistant strains of bacteria by atabrine. *Arch Biochem* 1964; **108**: 85–88.

(71) De Courcy SJ Jr, Sevag MG. Specificity and prevention of antibiotic resistance in Staphylococcus aureus. *Nature* 1966; **209**: 373–376.

(72) Sharda DC, Cornfeld D, Michie AJ. Effect of mepacrine (Atebrin) on the success of antibacterial treatment of urinary infections. *Arch Dis Child* 1966; **41**: 400–401.

(73) Horwitz MR, Eshleman JL, Sevag MG, De Courcy SJ Jr, Mudd S, Blakemore WS. Effect of combined atabrine-antimicrobial drug therapy on urinary tract infections: *in vitro* and *in vivo* studies. *Surg Forum* 1968; **19**: 532–534.

(74) Eshleman JL, Horwitz MR, De Courcy SJ Jr, Mudd S, Blakemore WS. Atabrine as an adjuvant in chemotherapy of urinary tract infections. *J Urol* 1970; **104**: 902–907.

(75) WHO Press Release. Drugs in pregnancy and at delivery, Nov. 12, 1984.